Atlas of Office-based Blue Laser Therapy in Laryngology

Abdul Latif Hamdan
Robert Thayer Sataloff
Mary J. Hawkshaw
Omar Ramadan

Atlas of Office-based Blue Laser Therapy in Laryngology

Springer

Abdul Latif Hamdan
Department of Otolaryngology- Head and Neck Surgery
American University of Beirut Medical Center
Beirut, Lebanon

Mary J. Hawkshaw
Department of Otolaryngology – Head and Neck Surgery
Drexel University College of Medicine
Philadelphia, PA, USA

Robert Thayer Sataloff
Department of Otolaryngology - Head and Neck Surgery
Drexel University College of Medicine
Philadelphia, PA, USA

Omar Ramadan
Department of Otolaryngology - Head and Neck Surgery
Drexel University College of Medicine
Philadelphia, PA, USA

ISBN 978-3-031-71824-3 ISBN 978-3-031-71825-0 (eBook)
https://doi.org/10.1007/978-3-031-71825-0

This Springer imprint is published by the registered company Springer Nature Switzerland AG
The registered company address is: Gewerbestrasse 11, 6330 Cham, Switzerland

To our families

Preface

Use of lasers in laryngology started in 1972 and has become increasingly common. It is safe and practical to use lasers not only in the operating room (OR) under anesthesia, but also in an office setting, eliminating much of the morbidity and expense associated with general anesthesia and surgery in an OR. Many advances have improved laser therapy, particularly introduction of the blue laser with a wavelength of 445 nm which became available in 2018. Like all other lasers, it has unique properties including melanin absorption characteristics which make it a slightly different from predecessor photoangiolytic lasers and which must be understood by a surgeon in order to achieve optimal results.

This *Atlas of Office-Based Blue Laser Therapy in Laryngology* offers readers with practical insights based on experience using blue laser in an office setting for a variety of otolaryngology conditions. Chapter 1 offers a brief historical overview of laser applications in laryngology. Chapter 2 reviews the techniques for applying topical anesthesia to the larynx in order to permit safe and comfortable in-office surgery. Chapter 3 reviews techniques for treating vocal fold polyps with blue laser in the office and presents the first of approximately 300 images and videos of office-based blue laser therapy. Chapter 4 discusses blue laser techniques for management of Reinke's edema, and Chap. 5 discusses how the laser should be handled for treatment of vocal fold cysts. Chapter 6 describes blue laser therapy for vascular lesions, one of the most common and effective uses of photoangiolytic laser therapy. Chapter 7 discusses how the laser can be used to treat vocal fold granulomas not only on the vocal process, but also elsewhere on the vocal fold. In some cases, it is appropriate to treat recurrent respiratory papillomatosis (RRP) in an office setting, and techniques specific to this application are presented in Chap. 8. Chapter 9 reviews in-office laser surgery for vocal fold leukoplakia, stressing the importance of biopsy and of appropriate selection of lesions for office-based laser therapy. In Chap. 10, the authors discuss less common uses of in-office laser therapy including treatment of bilateral vocal fold paralysis, lesions adjacent to the larynx, subglottic stenosis, and partial implant extrusion.

The authors hope that the illustrations, images and videos, and the discussions provided to share our clinical experience will prove useful to our colleagues, particularly relatively new users of blue laser therapy who might learn from our cases so that they do not have quite so long a learning curve and do not have to make the mistakes that we made when we first began using this new and excellent technology.

Beirut, Lebanon
Philadelphia, PA, USA

Abdul Latif Hamdan
Robert Thayer Sataloff
Mary J. Hawkshaw
Omar Ramadan

Acknowledgments

Special gratitude to Dr. Lana Ghzayel, Research Associate at the American University of Beirut Medical Center, for her valuable contribution and help in the review of this Atlas.

Contents

1 Introduction to Lasers in Laryngology . . . 1
1.1 Introduction . . . 1
References . . . 2

2 Topical Anesthesia to the Larynx . . . 3
2.1 Introduction . . . 3
References . . . 4

3 Office-Based Blue Laser Therapy for Vocal Fold Polyps . . . 7
3.1 Introduction . . . 7
3.2 Case Presentations . . . 7
3.2.1 Case 3.1 . . . 7
3.2.2 Case 3.2 . . . 7
3.2.3 Case 3.3 . . . 9
3.2.4 Case 3.4 . . . 10
3.2.5 Case 3.5 . . . 12
3.2.6 Case 3.6 . . . 12
3.2.7 Case 3.7 . . . 12
3.2.8 Case 3.8 . . . 13
3.2.9 Case 3.9 . . . 14
3.2.10 Case 3.10 . . . 15
3.2.11 Case 3.11 . . . 16
3.2.12 Case 12. . . . 18
References . . . 20

4 Office-Based Blue Laser Therapy for Vocal Fold Reinke's Edema . . . 23
4.1 Introduction . . . 23
4.2 Case Presentations . . . 23
4.2.1 Case 4.1 . . . 23
4.2.2 Case 4.2 . . . 24
4.2.3 Case 4.3 . . . 25
4.2.4 Case 4.4 . . . 25
4.2.5 Case 4.5 . . . 25
4.2.6 Case 4.6 . . . 27
4.2.7 Case 4.7 . . . 29
4.2.8 Case 4.8 . . . 30
4.2.9 Case 4.9 . . . 30

4.2.10 Case 4.10 31
4.2.11 Case 4.11 32
4.2.12 Case 4.12 33
4.2.13 Case 4.13 34
4.2.14 Case 4.14 35
4.2.15 Case 4.15 36
References 38

5 Office-Based Blue Laser Therapy for Vocal Fold Cysts 39
5.1 Introduction 39
5.2 Case Presentations 39
5.2.1 Case 5.1 39
5.2.2 Case 5.2 40
5.2.3 Case 5.3 42
5.2.4 Case 5.4 42
5.2.5 Case 5.5 42
5.2.6 Case 5.6 43
References 46

6 Office-Based Blue Laser Therapy of Vocal Fold Varices and Other Vascular Lesions 49
6.1 Introduction 49
6.2 Case Presentations 49
6.2.1 Case 6.1 49
6.2.2 Case 6.2 50
6.2.3 Case 6.3 50
6.2.4 Case 6.4 52
6.2.5 Case 6.5 53
6.2.6 Case 6.6 54
References 55

7 Office-Based Blue Laser Therapy for Vocal Fold Granuloma 57
7.1 Introduction 57
7.2 Case Presentations 57
7.2.1 Case 7.1 57
7.2.2 Case 7.2 58
7.2.3 Case 7.3 58
7.2.4 Case 7.4 60
References 61

8 Office-Based Blue Laser Therapy for Recurrent Respiratory Papillomatosis 63
8.1 Introduction 63
8.2 Case Presentations 63
8.2.1 Case 8.1 63
8.2.2 Case 8.2 63
8.2.3 Case 8.3 64
8.2.4 Case 8.4 66
References 68

9 Office-Based Blue Laser Therapy for Vocal Fold Leukoplakia . . . 69
9.1 Introduction . . . 69
9.2 Case Presentations . . . 69
9.2.1 Case 9.1 . . . 69
9.2.2 Case 9.2 . . . 70
9.2.3 Case 9.3 . . . 70
9.2.4 Case 9.4 . . . 71
9.2.5 Case 9.5 . . . 74
9.2.6 Case 9.6 . . . 74
References . . . 75

10 Rare Applications of Office-Based Blue Laser Therapy . . . 77
10.1 Introduction . . . 77
10.2 Case Presentation . . . 77
10.2.1 Case 10.1 . . . 77
10.2.2 Case 10.2 . . . 77
10.2.3 Case 10.3 . . . 78
10.2.4 Case 10.4 . . . 78
References . . . 81

Index . . . 83

1 Introduction to Lasers in Laryngology

1.1 Introduction

The use of lasers has revolutionized otolaryngology practice for decades. In 1972, the carbon dioxide (CO_2) laser (10.600 nm wavelength) was introduced in laryngology and has remained popular as a surgical tool in addition to cold instrumentation [1]. Its cutting and hemostatic properties allow excision and debulking of benign and malignant lesions of the larynx with minimal bleeding. When used in a focused mode, the CO2 laser acts as a hemostatic scalpel, whereas in the defocused mode it allows vaporization of tissues in a relatively bloodless manner [2–4]. The advances in spot size and in techniques of delivery using pulse and super-pulse modes have refined its use further resulting in minimal damage to the deep structures of the vocal folds and related scar. The thulium laser with a wavelength of 2013 nm is a less commonly used diode pumped solid laser. The thulium laser also targets chromophore of water with the additional benefit of being delivered via fibers of different sizes [5]. When used in near-contact mode, the thulium laser allows tangential cutting with hemostatic properties superior to the CO2 laser [6, 7]. A main limitation of the CO2 and thulium laser is tissue loss secondary to carbonization and excessive heating [4]. This has spurred the development of photoangiolytic lasers, initially, the pulse dye laser (PDL) with a wavelength of 585 nm, and the potassium titanyl phosphate (KTP) laser with a wavelength 532 nm wavelength. The photoangiolytic lasers target primarily oxyhemoglobin and not water. Their use for the treatment of vascular lesions of the vocal folds has reduced injury to the mucosal cover and underlying deep layers of the lamina propria [8–12]. The KTP laser gained popularity over the PDL partially because of its extended pulse width of 1.5 ms, which allows better hemostasis and minimal procedural bleeding. Other advantages of the KPT laser over the PDL include the smaller fiber size for delivery and the robust machine that is less prone to failure [13, 14].

In 2018, a new laser with a wavelength of 445 nm was introduced to the market [15]. The blue laser is a "hybrid" type of laser that combines the cutting properties of the diode lasers and the hemostatic properties of the photoangiolytic lasers. When used in the close-to-contact mode, it allows precise cutting and hemostatic dissection. Its photoangiolytic and cutting properties are based primarily on the distance from the glass fiber tip to the target tissue. Increasing that distance results in a decrease in energy absorption and divergence of the laser beam at a steady angle [14]. Another important variable is the speed with which the glass fiber is moved over the lesion during surgery. With an increase in the sideways movement of the glass fiber, there is a decrease in energy delivered and in tissue absorption. Blue laser also can be used in contact mode without damage to the fiber.

A. L. Hamdan et al., *Atlas of Office-based Blue Laser Therapy in Laryngology*,
https://doi.org/10.1007/978-3-031-71825-0_1

The evolution in laryngology practice toward office-based surgery over the last two decades has been accompanied by the use of lasers in the office with relatively good patient tolerance and surgical outcome [15–19]. With the different types of lasers available, the therapeutic armamentarium of laryngologists has increased markedly. In addition to the type of lasers to be selected, factors to consider in the choice of a laser is its wavelength, depth of absorption, extent of scattering, mode of delivery, and fiber size.

This book provides more than 300 images and video-recordings of office-based blue laser therapy for benign and premalignant lesions of the vocal folds and larynx. The authors hope that these examples will provide practice insights for surgeons and will serve as a source of various experience to help facilitate achievement of good outcomes with blue laser even when a surgeon is just beginning to adopt the instrument for in-office patient care.

References

1. Strong MS, Jako GI. Laser surgery in the larynx. Early clinical experience with continuous CO2 laser. Ann Otol Rhinol Laryngol. 1972;81:791–8.
2. Sataloff RT, Spiegel JR, Hawkshaw M, et al. Laser surgery of the larynx: the case for caution. Ear Nose Throat J. 1992;71(11):593–5.
3. Ekbom DC, Bayan SL, Goates AJ, et al. Endoscopic wedge excisions with CO2 laser for subglottic stenosis. Laryngoscope. 2021;131(4):E1062–6.
4. Benninger MS. Microdissection or microspot CO2 laser for limited vocal fold benign lesions: a prospective randomized trial. Laryngoscope. 2000;110(2 Pt 2 Suppl 92):1–17.
5. Zeitels SM, Burns JA. Office-based laryngeal laser surgery with local anesthesia. Curr Opin Otolaryngol Head Neck Surg. 2007;15(3):141–7.
6. Koufman JA, Rees CJ, Frazier WD, et al. Office-based laryngeal laser surgery: a review of 443 cases using three wavelengths. Otolaryngol Head Neck Surg. 2007;137(1):146–51.
7. Hamdan AL, Khalifee E, Ghanem A. Application of thulium laser as office-based procedure in patients with vocal fold polyps. J Voice. 2020;34(1):140–4.
8. McMillan K, Shapshay SM, McGilligan JA, et al. A 585-nanometer pulsed dye laser treatment of laryngeal papillomas: preliminary report. Laryngoscope. 1998;108(7):968–72.
9. Franco RA Jr, Farinelli WA, Zeitels SM, et al. 585-nm pulsed dye laser treatment of glottal papillomatosis. Ann Otol Rhinol Laryngol. 2002;111(6):486–92.
10. Burns JA, Zeitels SM, Akst LM, et al. 532 nm pulsed potassium-titanyl-phosphate laser treatment of laryngeal papillomatosis under general anesthesia. Laryngoscope. 2007;117(8):1500–4.
11. Sataloff RT. Voice surgery. In: Sataloff RT, editor. Professional voice: the science and art of clinical care. 4th ed. San Diego, CA: Plural Publishing; 2017. p. 1371–9.
12. Friedman AD, Hillman RE, Landau-Zemer T, et al. Voice outcomes for photoangiolytic KTP laser treatment of early glottic cancer. Ann Otol Rhinol Laryngol. 2013;122(3):151–8.
13. Zeitels SM, Burns JA, Lopez-Guerra G, et al. Photoangiolytic laser treatment of early glottic cancer: a new management strategy. Ann Otol Rhinol Laryngol Suppl. 2008;199:3–24.
14. Hess M, Fleischer S, Ernstberger M. New 445 nm blue laser for laryngeal surgery combines photoangiolytic and cutting properties. Eur Arch Otorrinolaringol. 2018;275(6):1557–67.
15. Woo P. Office-based laryngeal procedures. Rev Otolaryngol Clin North Am. 2006;39(1):111–33.
16. Hamdan AL, Jabbour C, Khalifee E, et al. Tolerance of patients using different approaches in laryngeal office-based procedures. J Voice. 2023;37(2):263–7.
17. Rees CJ, Halum SL, Wijewickrama RC, et al. Patient tolerance of in-office pulsed dye laser treatments to the upper aerodigestive tract. Otolaryngol Head Neck Surg. 2006;134(6):1023–7.
18. Hamdan AL, Sataloff RT, Hawkshaw MJ. Office-based laryngeal surgery. Springer Nature; 2022.
19. Hamdan AL, Sataloff RT, Ramadan O, Eichorn D, Hawkshaw MJ. Blue laser surgery in laryngology. Springer Nature; 2023.

2 Topical Anesthesia to the Larynx

2.1 Introduction

The use of topical anesthesia in surgery of the upper aerodigestive tract is not new. The first agent used in the nineteen century was cocaine, following which many synthetic anesthetics have been introduced [1]. Local anesthetics act by blocking the membranous sodium channels of sensory nerves thus inhibiting the initiation and propagation of action potentials. When applied to the laryngeal mucosa, this results in numbness and impaired sensation [2]. The main advantage of topical anesthesia to the upper aerodigestive tract, in addition to sparing the patient the risk of general anesthesia, is that it allows the surgeon to communicate with the patient who is awake during surgery. Engaging the patient by asking him or her to perform different phonatory and breathing tasks can facilitate surgery and help improve the surgical outcome [3, 4]. Although the application of topical anesthesia to the larynx and pharynx has enabled otolaryngologists to perform office-based laryngeal surgery safely, adverse events such as dyspnea and sensation of shortness of breath during surgery can occur. These are ascribed mostly to dysregulation in upper airway reflexes and alteration in airflow resistance. Another frequent complaint is delay in the ability to swallow due to impairment of oral and pharyngeal sensation [5, 6].

Topical anesthesia to the larynx can be delivered using different approaches: perioral, transcervical, and transnasal [7]. In the perioral approach, the anesthetic solution is instilled at the tip of the epiglottis and into the laryngeal inlet via a curved cannula while the tongue is held by the patient or the surgeon. The installation of the anesthetic solution can be made with or without an assistant holding a flexible nasopharyngoscope for visualization. In the transcervical approach, the anesthetic solution is injected percutaneously via a puncture into the trachea, cricothyroid membrane, or thyrohyoid membrane. It is important to check for air bubbles before injecting the local anesthetic, particularly when the injection is made without fiberoptic guidance. A cough is usually elicited which allows dispersion of the anesthetic solution into the larynx and pharynx. Very rarely, the cough associated with transtracheal injection can result in pneumomediastinum. A third approach to deliver the local anesthetic solution into the larynx is via the working channel of a flexible nasopharyngoscope with or without the use of a cannula. This approach is most advantageous in patients with a strong gag reflex and/or a narrow oropharyngeal cavity which impairs the use of the transoral approach. It is also advocated in patients with obscure anatomic cervical landmarks due to conditions such as obesity. The anesthetic solution is dripped on the vocal folds while the patient is asked to phonate, a technique referred to as "laryngeal gargle" (Video 2.1) [8].

Supplementary Information The online version contains supplementary material available at https://doi.org/10.1007/978-3-031-71825-0_2.

A. L. Hamdan et al., *Atlas of Office-based Blue Laser Therapy in Laryngology*,
https://doi.org/10.1007/978-3-031-71825-0_2

A less commonly performed technique to anesthetize the larynx is via the use of a nebulizer or atomizer. The use of a nebulizer was described first in 1964 by Erickson et al as an effective means to anesthetize the laryngeal mucosa [9]. In 1987, Thawley stressed its added value, namely the avoidance of laryngeal manipulation during the delivery of the anesthetic solution [10]. Another advantage of using a nebulizer is the even distribution of the anesthetic solution in the pharynx and larynx. However, its effectiveness is determined by the size of the particle that is delivered. Small particles tend to can reach the lower airway while large particles are more likely to deposit on the vocal folds and other laryngeal structures. The efficacy of nebulized anesthesia is very high reaching up to 96% in some cases. Christoforidis et al advocated the use of ultrasonic nebulizer to control better the particle size and hence the even distribution of the anesthetic [11]. Another method that is used rarely in the office setting to anesthetize the laryngopharyngeal complex is superior laryngeal nerve block. This method involves injecting lidocaine solution at the entry point of the internal branch of the superior laryngeal nerve between the superior cornu of the thyroid cartilage and the greater cornu of the hyoid bone. Superior laryngeal nerve block usually is reserved for those who fail other routes of administration of local anesthetics [12], or for patients with a particular strong gag reflex who have a compelling need for awake in-office surgery.

Although each method of application of local anesthesia to the larynx and pharynx has its unique advantages, the superiority of one method over another has not been established [8, 13]. The choice of method is based on many factors that can be patient-related and/or physician-related. Patient-related factors include the anatomy of the neck, severity of gag reflex, and patient's tolerance. Physician-related factors include the level of dexterity/agility of the physician and his or her personal preference. Another possible limitation to the use of one method versus another is the availability or lack of resources such as the type of equipment and instrumentation needed.

Despite the well-established safety of topical anesthesia to the upper airway in an office setting, the risk of systemic toxicity should not be overlooked [14, 15]. Although it is rare, systemic toxicity may occur if a high dose of an anesthetic solution has been given. When lidocaine is used, the dose should not exceed 4.5 mg/kg in order to avoid adverse systemic events. Other factors to consider are the variation in the absorption rate of different local anesthetics and the time interval between anesthesia administrations. Symptoms such as confusion, headache, and tinnitus should alert the physician to the neurologic toxic reaction. Hemodynamic changes such as bradycardia and hypotension are also alarming signs of cardiovascular toxicity that should prompt the treating physician to intervene promptly [16, 17]. Methemoglobinemia characterized by oxidation of hemoglobin is extremely rare but carries a significant morbidity should it occur and needs to be addressed urgently using methylene blue [18].

References

1. Jourdy DN, Kacker A. Regional anesthesia for office-based procedures in otorhinolaryngology. Anesthesiol Clin. 2010;28(3):457–68.
2. Simpson CB, Amin MR, Postma GN. Topical anesthesia of the airway and esophagus. Ear Nose Throat J. 2004;83(7 Suppl 2):2–5.
3. Hamdan AL, Sataloff RT, Hawkshaw MJ. Topical anesthesia in office-based laryngeal surgery. In: Hamdan AL, Sataloff RT, Hawkshaw MJ, editors. Office-based laryngeal surgery. Springer Nature; 2022.
4. Sulica L, Blitzer A. Anesthesia for laryngeal surgery in the office. Laryngoscope. 2000;110(10 Pt 1):1777–9.
5. Raphael JH, Stanley GD, Langton JA. Effects of topical benzocaine and lignocaine on upper airway reflex sensitivity. Anaesthesia. 1996;51(2):114–8.
6. Liistro G, Stănescu DC, Veriter C, et al. Upper airway anesthesia induces airflow limitation in awake humans. Surv Anesthesiol. 1993;37(3):131.
7. Wellenstein DJ, Van der Wal RAB, Schutte HW, et al. Topical anesthesia for endoscopic office-based procedures of the upper aerodigestive tract. J Voice. 2019;33(5):732–46.
8. Woo P. Office-based laryngeal procedures. Otolaryngol Clin N Am. 2006;39(1):111–33.
9. Erickson JC 3rd. Surface anesthesia of the airway and larynx. Int Anesthesiol Clin. 1964;2(3):709–24.

10. Thawley SE. Nebulized anesthesia for the nose, pharynx, larynx, and trachea. Laryngoscope. 1987;97(4):499–500.
11. Christoforidis AJ, Tomashefski JF, Mitchell RI. Use of an ultrasonic nebulizer for the application of oropharyngeal, laryngeal and tracheobronchial anesthesia. Chest. 1971;59(6):629–33.
12. Gotta AW, Sullivan CA. Anesthesia of the upper airway using topical anesthetic and superior laryngeal nerve block. Br J Anaesth. 1981;53(10):1055–8.
13. Hamdan AL, Jabbour C, Khalifee E, et al. Tolerance of patients using different approaches in laryngeal office-based procedures. J Voice. 2023;37(2):263–7.
14. Postma GN, Cohen JT, Belafsky PC, et al. Transnasal esophagoscopy: revisited (over 700 consecutive cases). Laryngoscope. 2005;115(2):321–3.
15. Sulica L, Rosen CA, Postma GN, et al. Current practice in injection augmentation of the vocal folds: indications, treatment principles, techniques, and complications. Laryngoscope. 2010;120(2):319–25.
16. Macfarlane AJR, Gitman M, Bornstein KJ, et al. Updates in our understanding of local anaesthetic systemic toxicity: a narrative review. Anaesthesia. 2021;76 Suppl 1(S1):27–39.
17. Wadlund DL. Local anesthetic systemic toxicity. AORN J. 2017;106(5):367–77.
18. Hieger MA, Afeld JL, Cumpston KL, et al. Topical benzocaine and methemoglobinemia. Am J Ther. 2017;24(5):e596.

3 Office-Based Blue Laser Therapy for Vocal Fold Polyps

3.1 Introduction

Vocal fold polyps are benign lesions of the vocal folds commonly encountered in men. The etiology is multifaceted with phonotrauma being a common cause [1, 2]. Other risk factors include laryngopharyngeal reflux disease, the use of anticoagulants, vocal fold paresis, and vocal fold structural abnormalities [3, 4]. Patients usually present with a change in voice quality and an increase in phonatory effort. On laryngeal examination, the lesion can be gelatinous, or angiomatous or fibrotic, and is found most commonly at the middle or anterior one third of the vocal fold. Surgical excision is usually recommended with preoperative and postoperative voice therapy for the management of associated tension in the laryngeal muscles [5, 6]. Office-based laser therapy has gained popularity as an alternative treatment to surgical excision in the operating room, particularly in patients with high risk for general anesthesia [7, 8]. Various types of lasers are used including the blue laser with a wavelength of 445 nm [9, 10]. This chapter presents cases of vocal fold polyp treated in-office using the blue laser. Preoperative, intraoperative, and postoperative images with video-recordings of the surgical technique help illustrate principles and techniques.

Supplementary Information The online version contains supplementary material available at https://doi.org/10.1007/978-3-031-71825-0_3.

3.2 Case Presentations

3.2.1 Case 3.1

A 40-year-old male, smoker, presented to the Voice Clinic (ALH) with hoarseness of a few months' duration. The patient denied any history of voice abuse, allergy, or reflux disease. His Voice Handicap Index (VHI-10) score was 25. Aerodynamic analysis showed a maximum phonation time (MPT) of 6.7 seconds. Laryngeal examination revealed a right vocal fold hemorrhagic polyp with a reactive lesion on the left vocal fold (Fig. 3.1a). The patient underwent office-based blue laser therapy for his right vocal fold polyp using the 400 micrometers glass fiber (power 10 ms, pulse duration 10 ms, and pause time 300 ms) (Fig. 3.1b and c; Video 3.1). The procedure was tolerated well by the patient without any complications. On follow-up 2 months later, the patient reported improvement in his voice quality. His VHI-10 score dropped to 0. There was an increase in the MPT to 13 seconds. Laryngeal examination showed complete regression of the disease (Fig. 3.1d).

3.2.2 Case 3.2

A 47-year-old woman presented to the Voice Clinic (ALH) with a 2–3 month history of hoarseness following a COVID-19 infection. The patient denied any history of smoking, voice

A. L. Hamdan et al., *Atlas of Office-based Blue Laser Therapy in Laryngology*,
https://doi.org/10.1007/978-3-031-71825-0_3

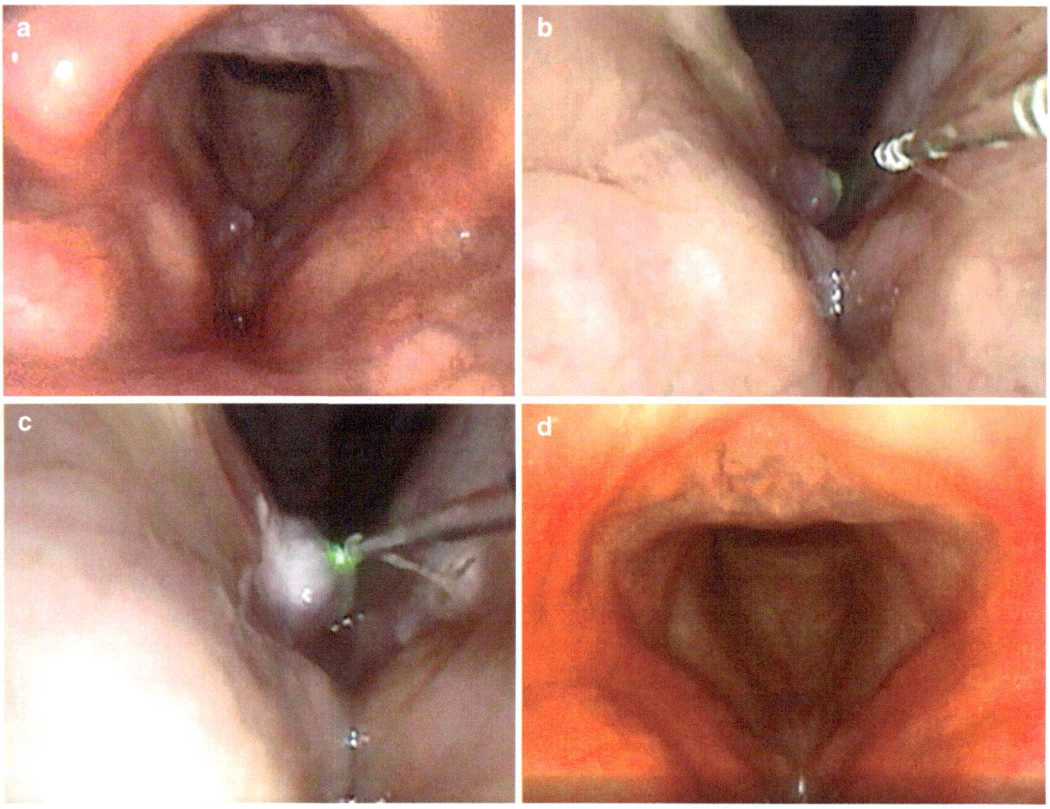

Fig. 3.1 (**a**) An endoscopic view of the larynx showing a hemorrhagic polyp at the anterior one third of the right vocal fold, with mild submucosal hemorrhage. Note the reactive lesion on the left vocal fold opposite to the polyp. (**b**) An intraoperative view of the larynx showing the blue laser glass fiber in noncontact mode aiming at the lesion. (**c**) An endoscopic view of the larynx showing the blue laser in contact with the right vocal fold polyp. Note the aberrant laser strikes on the left vocal fold. (**d**) A view of the larynx 2 months after surgery showing complete regression of the lesion

abuse, allergy, or reflux disease. Her Voice Handicap Index (VHI-10) score at presentation was 20. Acoustic analysis showed a fundamental frequency (F0) of 208.9 Hz, habitual pitch (HP) of 181.4 Hz, jitter 2.21, shimmer 9.02, a noise-to-harmonic ratio (NHR) of 0.12, and a voice turbulence index (VTI) of 0.045. Her maximum phonation time (MPT) was 10.15 seconds. Laryngeal endoscopic examination revealed a left vocal fold hemorrhagic polyp with yellowish discoloration of the upper surface of the vocal fold suggestive of a resolving hematoma (Fig. 3.2a). The patient underwent office-based blue laser therapy for the left vocal fold hemorrhagic polyp using contact and noncontact modes (Fig. 3.2b and c; Video 3.2). Following laser therapy, 0.2 ml of dexamethasone (8 mg/2 ml) was injected into the surgical bed using a 25-gauge needle that was introduced through the working channel of the flexible laryngoscope. The procedure was tolerated well by the patient with no complications noted. On follow-up 2 months later, the patient had marked improvement in her voice quality. Her VHI-10 score dropped to 0. Acoustic analysis showed a decrease in shimmer to 2.14 and a slight increase in the F0 to 211.5. Laryngeal examination revealed complete regression of the lesion (Fig. 3.2d).

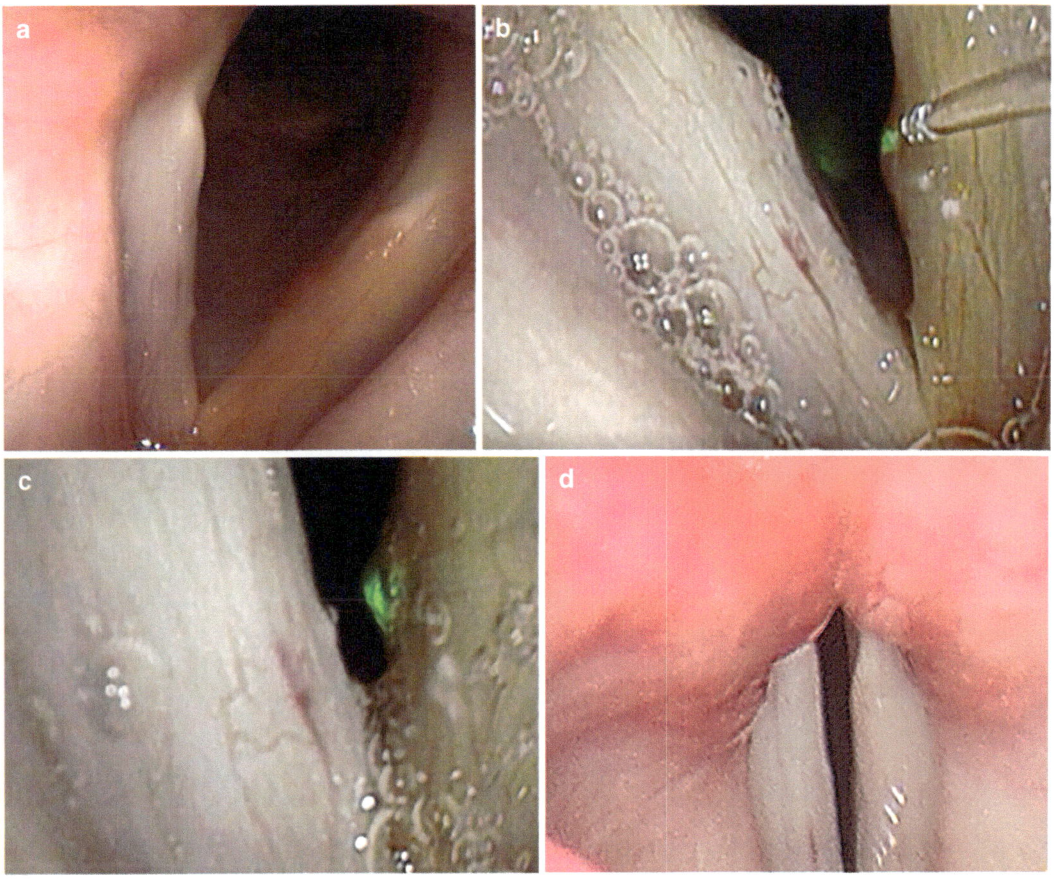

Fig. 3.2 (**a**) An endoscopic view of the larynx showing a left vocal fold hemorrhagic polyp with yellowish discoloration of the upper surface of the left vocal fold suggestive of a submucosal hematoma that was resolving. Note the dilated vessels on the right vocal fold running parallel to the free margin. (**b**) An endoscopic view of the larynx showing the blue laser glass fiber used in noncontact mode. (**c**) An endoscopic view showing the blue laser glass fiber in contact with the left vocal fold polyp. (**d**) A view of the larynx 2 months following laser therapy showing complete regression of the lesion

3.2.3 Case 3.3

A 42-year-old man presented to the Voice Clinic (ALH) with hoarseness of a few months' duration. The patient had a history of voice abuse and reflux disease but denied any history of smoking or allergy. His Voice Handicap Index (VHI-10) score was 24. Acoustic analysis showed a fundamental frequency (F0) of 117 Hz, habitual pitch (HP) of 135.16 Hz, jitter 1.07, shimmer 4.9, a noise-to-harmonic ratio (NHR) of 0.152 and a voice turbulence index (VTI) of 0.033. Aerodynamic analysis showed a maximum phonation time (MPT) of 10.43 seconds. Laryngeal flexible endoscopy revealed a left vocal fold hemorrhagic polyp and a reactive lesion on the right vocal fold opposite to the polyp (Fig. 3.3a). The patient underwent office-based blue laser therapy for the left vocal fold polyp using the 400-micrometer glass fiber in contact and noncontact modes (Fig. 3.3b and c; Video 3.3). A total of 55.6 Joules was delivered. Following laser therapy, 0.2 ml of dexamethasone (8 mg/2 ml) was injected into each vocal fold.

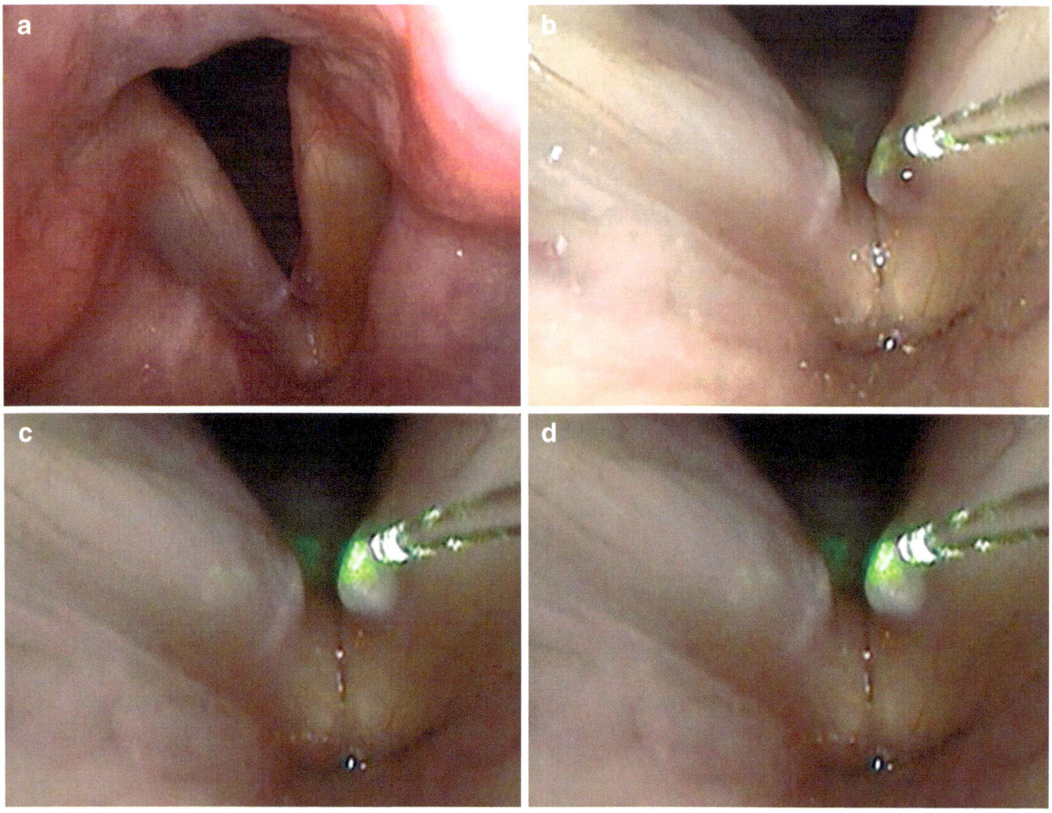

Fig. 3.3 (**a**) A endoscopic view of the larynx showing left vocal fold polyp and a reactive lesion on the right vocal fold. Note the yellowish discoloration of the left vocal fold suggestive of a resolving hematoma. (**b**) An endoscopic view of the larynx showing the blue laser glass fiber in noncontact mode. (**c**) An endoscopic view showing the blue laser glass fiber used in near contact mode against the left vocal fold polyp. Note the aberrant laser strikes on the right vocal fold. (**d**) A view of the larynx 4 weeks following laser therapy showing complete regression of the lesion. Note the presence of mild redness at the site of the surgery

The procedure was tolerated well by the patient with no complications. On follow-up 4 weeks later, the patient had marked improvement in his voice quality. His VHI-10 score dropped to 4. Acoustic analysis showed an increase in the F0 to 126.5 Hz and a decrease in the HP to 114.88 Hz. There was an increase in the MPT to 17 seconds. Laryngeal examination revealed complete regression of the lesion. Mild residual inflammation at the site of the surgery was noted (Fig. 3.3d).

3.2.4 Case 3.4

A 34-year-old female, heavy smoker, presented to the Voice Clinic (ALH) with hoarseness of a few months' duration. The patient had a history of voice abuse and reflux disease and denied any history of allergy. Her Voice Handicap Index (VHI-10) score was 33. Laryngeal flexible endoscopic examination revealed a large hemorrhagic polyp on the right vocal fold with submucosal hemorrhage. There were also irregular edematous changes on the free edge of the left vocal fold (Fig. 3.4a). A short course of steroid (40 mg of prednisone per day for a total of 10 days) was prescribed and she was advised complete voice rest for 5–7 days. On follow-up there was a decrease in the right vocal fold submucosal hemorrhage and edema with persistence of the polyp (Fig. 3.4b). The patient underwent office-based blue laser therapy for her right vocal fold lesion under local anesthesia and received a total of 71.7 J (Fig. 3.4c and d). Laser therapy

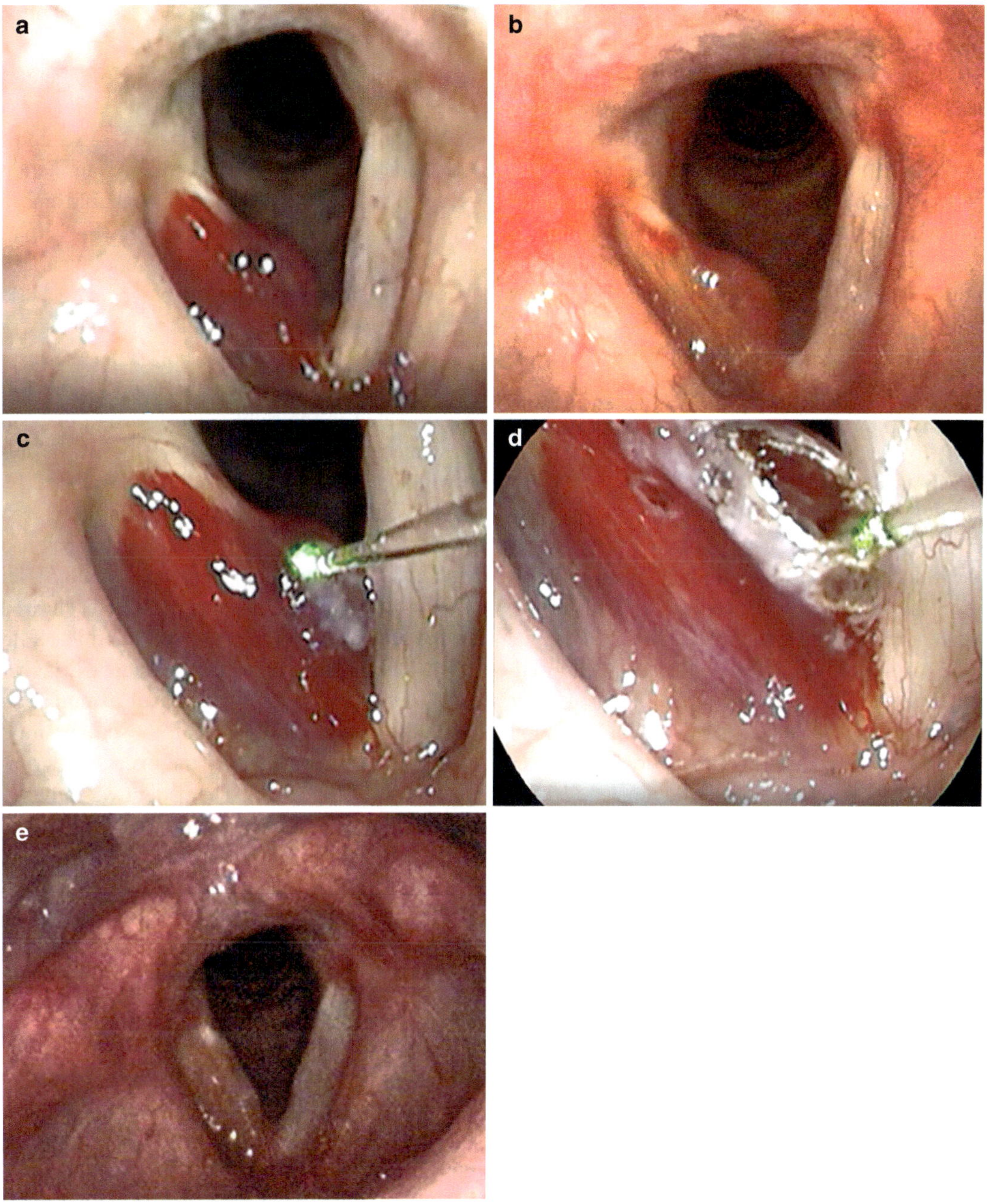

Fig. 3.4 (**a**) An endoscopic view of the larynx on presentation showing a right vocal fold sessile hemorrhagic polyp with submucosal hemorrhage involving the nearly entire musculomembranous vocal fold. (**b**) An endoscopic view of the larynx 10 days following medical treatment and voice rest showing a decrease in the submucosal hemorrhage and edema. Note the persistence of the hemorrhagic polyp on the right side. (**c**) An endoscopic view of the larynx during surgery showing the blue laser in non-contact mode. Note blanching of the lesion at the site of the laser beam. (**d**) Another intraoperative view showing the blue laser used in contact mode to incise the mucosal cover of the large polyp. (**e**) An endoscopic view of the larynx 5 weeks following surgery showing almost complete regression of the right vocal fold hemorrhage except for mild edema. Note the residual yellowish discoloration of the right vocal fold

was followed by an injection of 0.1 ml of dexamethasone (8 mg in 2 ml) into the right vocal fold and 0.1 ml into the left vocal fold. The procedure was tolerated well with no complications noted. On follow-up 5 weeks later, the patient reported marked improvement in her voice quality. Her VHI-10 score dropped to 8. Laryngeal endoscopic examination showed essentially complete regression of the right vocal fold hemorrhagic polyp with only residual edema noted at the surgical bed (Fig. 3.4e). The patient was reassured and advised to undergo steroid injection for the residual edema in her vocal fold.

3.2.5 Case 3.5

A 45-year-old male, heavy smoker, presented to the Voice Clinic (ALH) with hoarseness of a few months' duration. The patient had a history of voice abuse and denied any history of allergy or reflux disease. His Voice Handicap Index (VHI-10) score was 22. Laryngeal flexible endoscopic examination revealed a right vocal fold hemorrhagic polyp associated with signs of submucosal hemorrhage (Fig. 3.5a). Following a 10-day period of voice rest, the patient underwent office-based blue laser therapy (Fig. 3.5b and c). After the laser therapy, 0.2 ml of dexamethasone (8 mg/2 ml) was injected into each vocal fold using the 25-gauge flexible needle. The procedure was well tolerated by the patient with no complications noted.

On follow-up 4 weeks later, the patient reported marked improvement in his voice quality. His VHI-10 score dropped to 4. Laryngeal examination revealed partial regression in the size of the lesion (Fig. 3.5d).

3.2.6 Case 3.6

A 47-year-old female, heavy smoker, presented to the Voice Clinic (ALH) with intermittent hoarseness. The patient had a history of voice abuse and denied any history of allergy or reflux disease. Her Voice Handicap Index (VHI-10) score was 9. Acoustic analysis showed a fundamental frequency (F0) of 166.9 Hz, habitual pitch (HP) of 148.26 Hz, jitter 1.61, shimmer 3.85, noise-to-harmonic ratio (NHR) of 0.127, and a voice-turbulence-index (VTI) of 0.043. Her maximum phonation time (MPT) was 11.28 seconds. Laryngeal flexible endoscopic examination revealed a polyp on the right vocal fold and a reactive lesion on the left vocal fold (Fig. 3.6a). The patient underwent office-based blue laser therapy for the right vocal fold polyp using a 400 micrometer glass fiber. A total of 85 Joules was delivered (Fig. 3.6b and c). Following the laser therapy, 0.35 ml of dexamethasone (8 mg/2 ml) was injected in the right vocal fold and 0.25 ml was injected into the reactive lesion in the left vocal fold. The procedure was tolerated well by the patient without any complications.

On follow-up 6 weeks later, the patient had marked improvement in her voice quality. Her VHI-10 dropped to 3. Acoustic analysis showed an increase in the F0 to 188.75 Hz and in HP to 170.64 Hz. There was also an increase in her MPT to 25.19 seconds. Laryngeal examination revealed partial regression of the polyp, mild edema of both vocal folds, and excessive laryngeal tension (Fig. 3.6d). The patient was advised to undergo voice therapy to reduce the laryngeal tension.

3.2.7 Case 3.7

A 29-year-old man presented to the Voice Clinic with a change in voice quality of a few months' duration. The patient was a heavy smoker but he denied any history of reflux disease or allergy. His Voice Handicap Index-10 (VHI-10) score at presentation was 26. On perceptual evaluation, he had grade 2 dysphonia, grade 2 roughness, grade 1 breathiness, grade 0 asthenia, and grade 0 strain. Acoustic analysis showed a fundamental frequency (F_0) of 137.02 Hz, habitual pitch (HP) of 152.8 Hz, jitter 3.24, shimmer 12.61, noise-to-harmonic ratio (NHR) of 0.151, and voice turbulence index (VTI) of 0.093. His maximum phonation time (MPT) was 6.52 seconds. On laryngeal examination, he had a right anterior vocal fold polyp with a reactive lesion on the

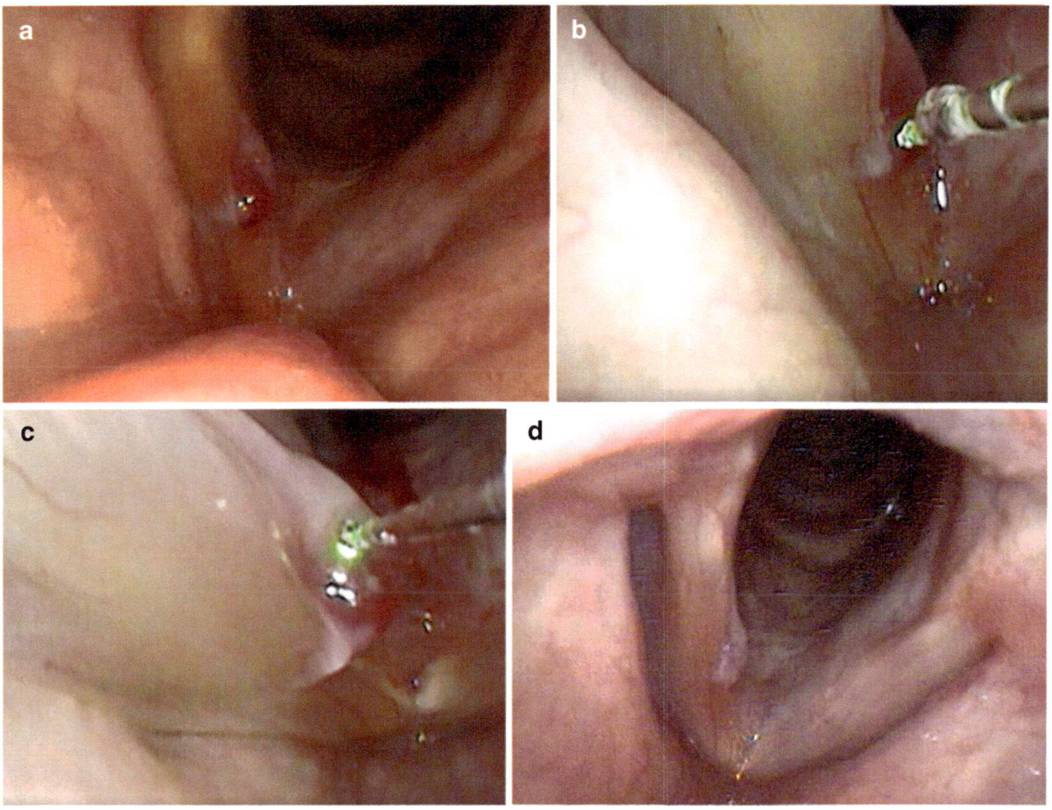

Fig. 3.5 (**a**) A preoperative view showing right vocal fold sessile hemorrhagic polyp with submucosal hemorrhage involving nearly the entire musculomembranous vocal fold. (**b**) An endoscopic view of the larynx showing the blue laser in noncontact mode. Note blanching of the lesion at the site of the laser beam. (**c**) Another intraoperative view of the vocal folds showing the blue laser used in contact mode against the right vocal fold polyp. (**d**) An endoscopic view of the larynx 4 weeks after surgery showing partial regression of the right vocal fold hemorrhagic polyp. Note blanching of the residual mass

opposite side (Fig. 3.7a). The patient underwent office-based blue laser therapy and received a total of 64.7 Joules. The laser therapy was followed by steroid injection into the right vocal fold (0.1 ml of dexamethasone 8 mg/2 ml) (Fig. 3.7b and c; Video 3.4). The lesion was ablated completely. On follow up 6 weeks later, the patient had marked improvement in his voice quality.

3.2.8 Case 3.8

A 78-year-old male, smoker, presented to the Voice Clinic (ALH) with hoarseness of a few weeks' duration. The patient had no symptoms related to breathing or swallowing, and he denied any history of reflux disease or allergy. His Voice Handicap Index-10 (VHI-10) score on presentation was 14. Acoustic analysis showed a fundamental frequency (F_0) of 126.85 Hz, habitual pitch (HP) of 152.68 Hz, jitter: 1.33, shimmer 3.32, noise-to-harmonic ratio (NHR) of 0.126, and voice turbulence index (VTI) of 0.056. His maximum phonation time (MPT) was 7.49 seconds. On laryngeal examination, he had a right vocal fold polypoid lesion with a reactive lesion on the left vocal fold (Fig. 3.8a). The patient underwent office-based blue laser therapy for both vocal fold lesions using power 10 watts, pulse duration 10 ms, and pulse pause 300 ms. A total of 40.8 Joules was given during the proce-

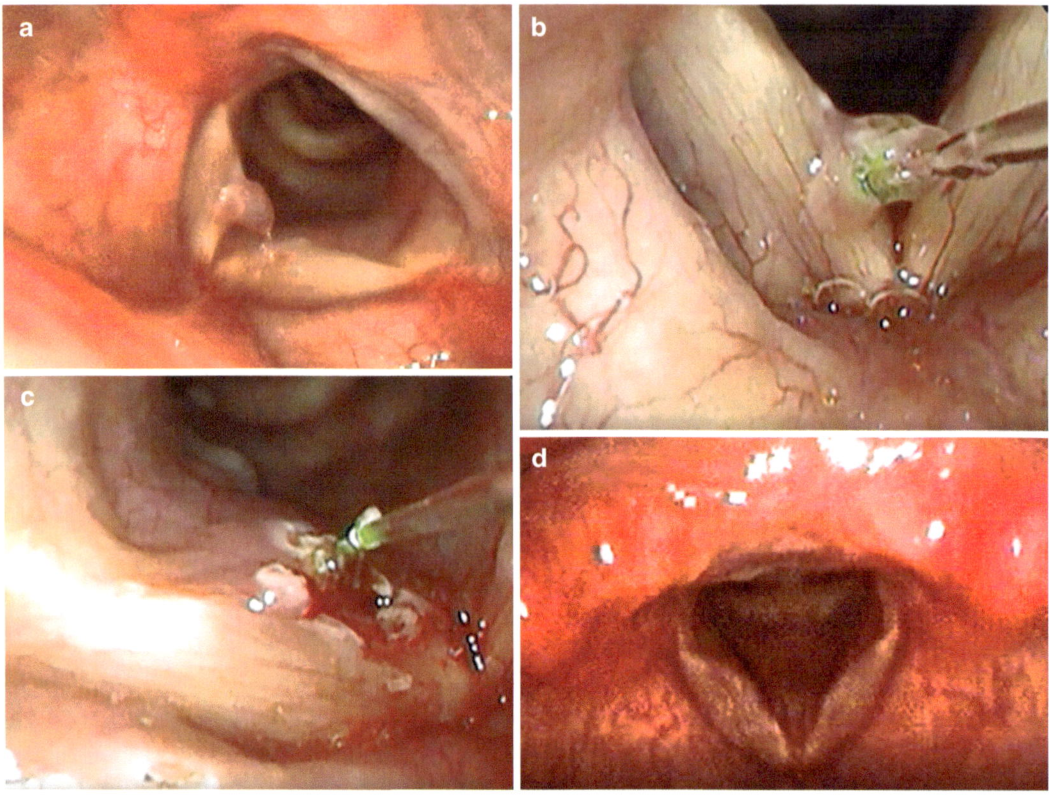

Fig. 3.6 (**a**) An endoscopic view of the larynx showing a pedunculated right vocal fold polyp. Note the localized edema and redness on the left vocal fold opposite to the lesion. (**b**) An intraoperative view of the larynx showing the tip of the blue laser glass fiber inserted into the right vocal fold polyp. (**c**) An endoscopic view of the larynx toward the end of surgery showing the surgical bed following laser therapy. (**d**) An endoscopic view of the larynx 6 weeks post-surgery showing partial regression of the lesion

dure (Fig. 3.8b). Two weeks after the surgery, the patient presented with marked improvement in his voice quality. Laryngeal endoscopic examination showed complete regression of both lesions. There was mild residual edema and redness in the surgical bed (Fig. 3.8c). The patient was advised on vocal hygiene therapy.

3.2.9 Case 3.9

A 40-year-old male, heavy smoker, presented to the Voice Clinic with hoarseness of few months' duration. The patient had a positive history of voice abuse and denied any history of allergy or reflux disease. His Voice Handicap Index-10 (VHI-10) score was 10. Acoustic analysis showed a fundamental frequency (F_0) of 104.6 Hz, habitual pitch (HP) of 90.1 Hz, jitter 0.76, shimmer 2.5, noise-to-harmonics ratio (NHR) of 0.137, and voice turbulence index (VTI) of 0.041. Aerodynamic analysis showed a maximum phonation time (MPT) of 21.54 seconds. Laryngeal endoscopic examination revealed a right vocal fold hemorrhagic polyp (Fig. 3.9a).

The patient underwent office-based blue laser therapy for the right vocal fold polyp using contact and noncontact modes, and a total of 92 Joules was delivered (Fig. 3.9b and c; Video 3.5). Residual polyp was removed completely using the cup-forceps (Fig. 3.9d). Following the laser

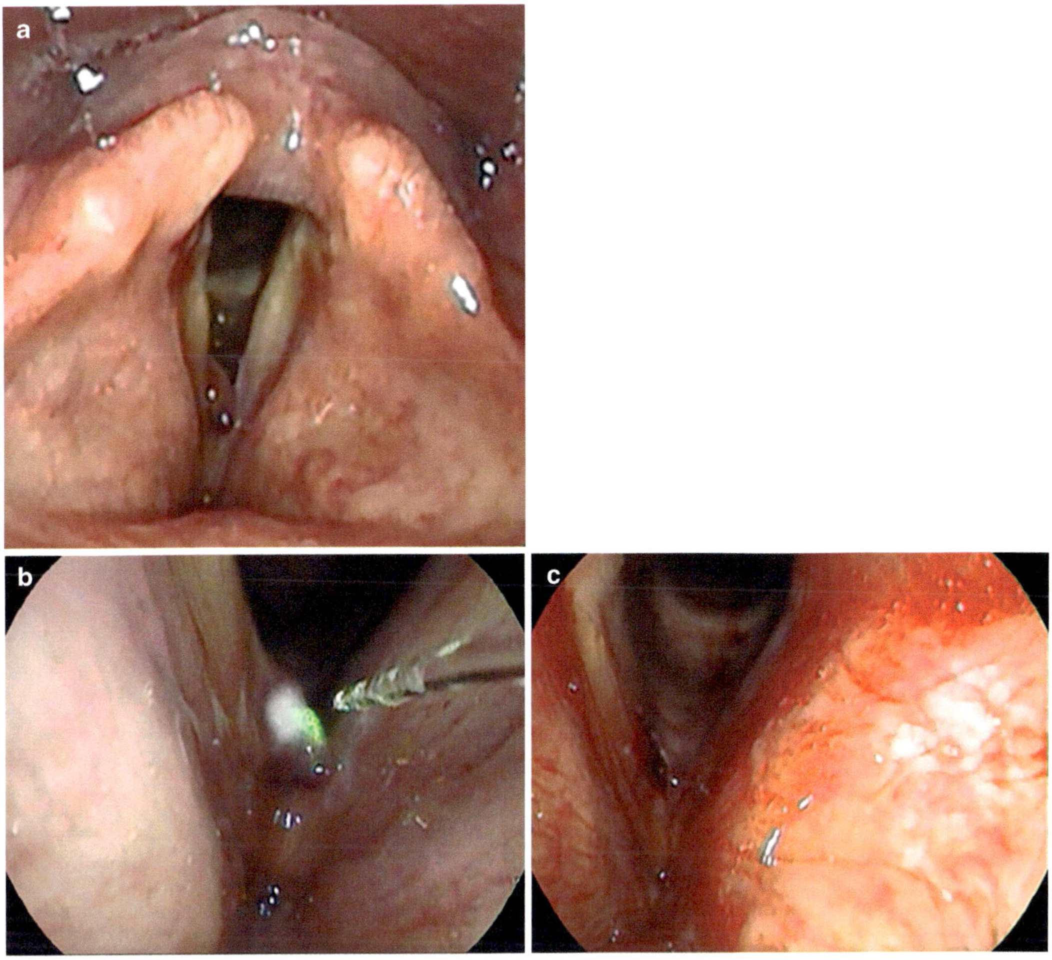

Fig. 3.7 (a) An endoscopic view of the larynx showing a right vocal fold hemorrhagic polyp. (b) An intraoperative view showing blanching of the right vocal fold polyp during the blue laser therapy. (c) A view of the larynx toward the end of the laser session. Note complete disappearance of the lesion

therapy, 0.4 ml of dexamethasone (8 mg/2 ml) was injected into the right vocal fold, and 0.1 cc was injected into the left vocal fold using a 25-gauge flexible needle (Fig. 3.9e). The procedure was tolerated well by the patient with no complications noted.

On follow-up 6 weeks later, the patient had marked improvement in his voice quality. His VHI-10 score dropped to 1. There was a decrease in the F_0 to 94.57 Hz, in HP to 86.9 Hz, in jitter to 0.21, and in shimmer to 1.13. There was an increase in the MPT to 29.6 seconds. Laryngeal endoscopic examination revealed complete regression of the lesion (Fig. 3.9f).

3.2.10 Case 3.10

A 68-year-old female, former smoker, presented to the voice clinic with hoarseness of a few months' duration. The patient denied any history of voice abuse, allergy, or reflux disease. Her Voice Handicap Index-10 (VHI-10) score was 6. Acoustic analysis showed a fundamental frequency (F0) of 165.5 Hz, habitual pitch (HP) of 151.42 Hz, jitter 1, shimmer 3.26, a noise-to-harmonics ratio (NHR) of 0.132, and voice to turbulence index (VTI) 0.033. Aerodynamic parameters revealed a maximum phonation time (MPT) of 7.4 seconds. Laryngeal endoscopic

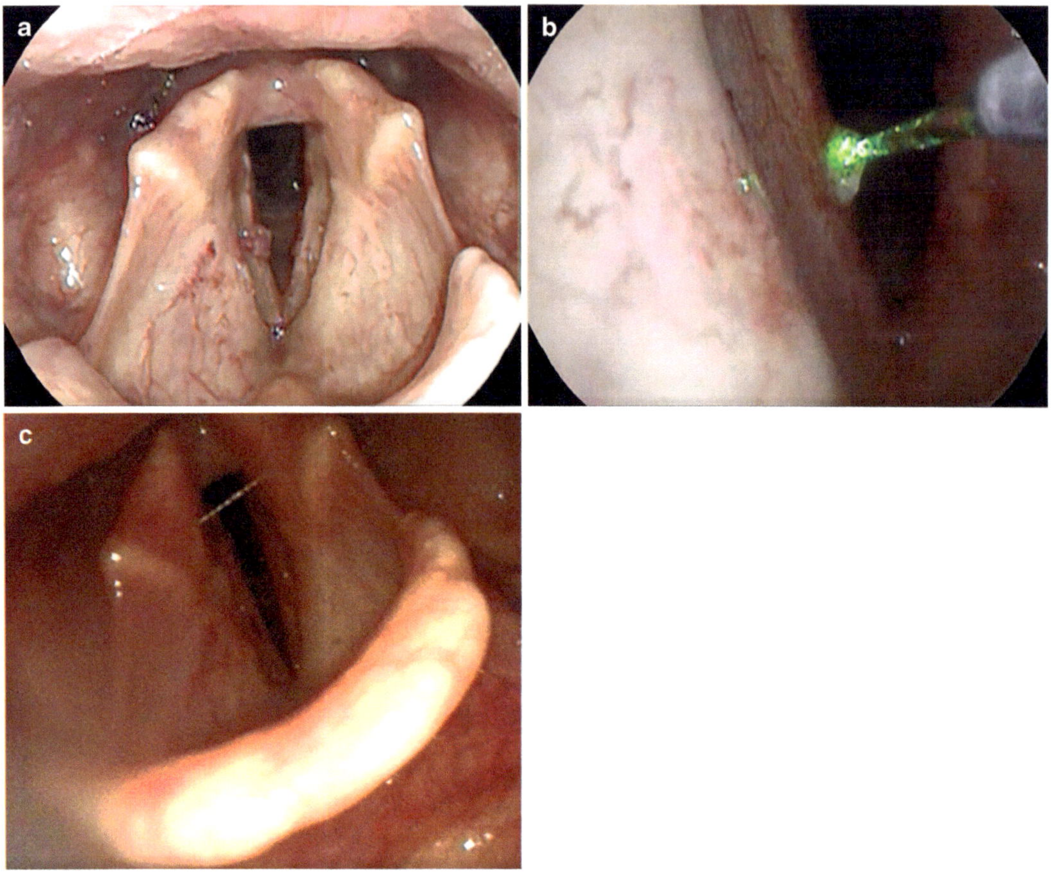

Fig. 3.8 (**a**) Laryngeal examination showing the polypod mass on the right vocal fold with a reactive lesion on the opposite vocal fold. (**b**) An endoscopic view of the larynx showing the blue laser glass fiber in contact with the polypoid lesion. (**c**) Postoperative view 3 weeks later showing complete regression of the lesion. Note the dilated vessel at the upper surface of the right vocal fold

examination revealed a right vocal fold hemorrhagic polyp (Fig. 3.10a). The patient underwent office-based blue laser therapy under local anesthesia (Fig. 3.10b–d; Video 3.6). The cup forceps was then used to eliminate residual polyp at the surgical site. Following the laser therapy, 0.1 ml of dexamethasone (8 mg/2 ml) was injected into each vocal folds. The procedure was tolerated well by the patient with no significant complications noted.

3.2.11 Case 3.11

A 60-year-old man presented to the Voice Clinic (ALH) with history of hoarseness for a few months. The patient is a former smoker and denied any history of voice abuse, allergy, or reflux disease. His Voice Handicap Index-10 (VHI-10) score was 12. Acoustic analysis showed a fundamental frequency (F0) of 196.68 Hz, a habitual pitch (HP) of 176.5 Hz, jitter 1.94, shimmer 6.78, a noise-to-harmonics ratio (NHR) of 0.15, and a voice to turbulence index (VTI) of 0.1. Aerodynamic analysis showed a maximum phonation time (MPT) of 8 seconds. Laryngeal flexible endoscopic examination revealed a hemorrhagic polyp on the left vocal fold and a reactive lesion on the right vocal fold (Fig. 3.11a).

The patient underwent office-based blue laser therapy using the contact and noncontact modes. A total of 80 Joules was delivered to the left vocal fold, and 10 Joules were delivered to the right

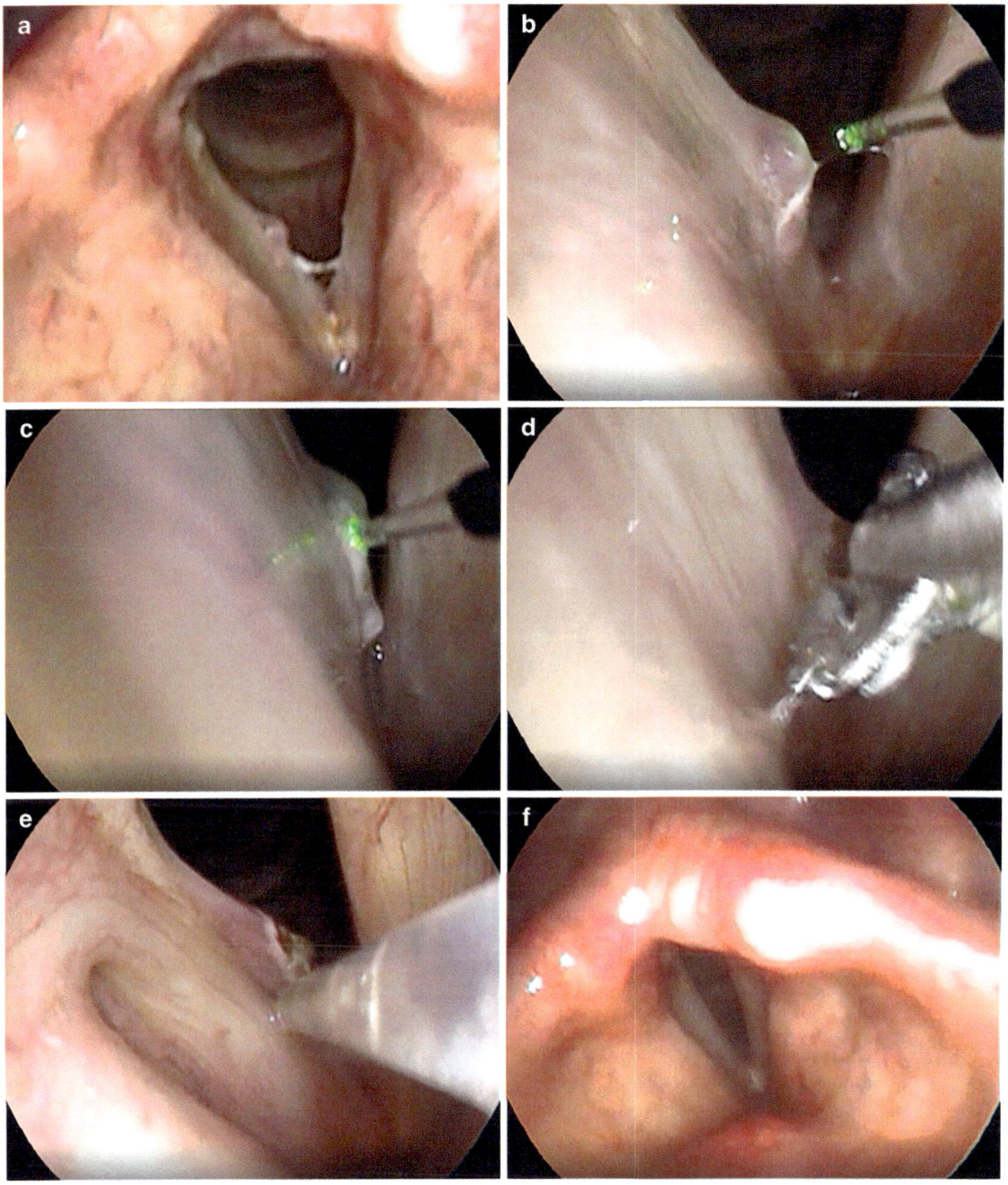

Fig. 3.9 (**a**) An endoscopic view of the larynx showing right vocal fold hemorrhagic polyp. (**b**) An intraoperative view of the larynx showing the blue laser beam aiming at the right vocal fold polyp. (**c**) An endoscopic view of the larynx showing the blue laser glass fiber in contact mode against the right vocal fold polyp. (**d**) An endoscopic view of the larynx toward the end of surgery showing removal of the surgical debris using a cup forceps. (**e**) An endoscopic view of the larynx showing steroid injection at the surgical bed (0.2 ml of dexamethasone 8 mg/2 ml). (**f**) Laryngeal examination 6 weeks after surgery showing complete regression of the lesion

vocal fold (Fig. 3.11a–f). A cup forceps was used to remove the remaining of the lesion (Fig. 3.11g). Following laser therapy, 1.5 ml of dexamethasone (8 mg/2 ml) was injected into the left vocal fold, and 1.5 ml was injected into the reactive lesion of the right vocal fold (Fig. 3.11h). The procedure was tolerated well by the patient with no complications noted.

3.2.12 Case 12

An 85-year-old male with history of multiple cardiac morbidities presented to our office (RTS) with dysphonia caused by a right vocal fold mass (Fig. 3.12a). He had a history of recurrent laryngeal leukoplakia treated with surgical removal. Due to his multiple comorbidities, we elected to vaporize the mass with the adjacent leukoplakia with blue laser (Fig. 3.12b). Six months after the procedure, there was complete regression of the mass and no recurrent leukoplakia (Fig. 3.12c).

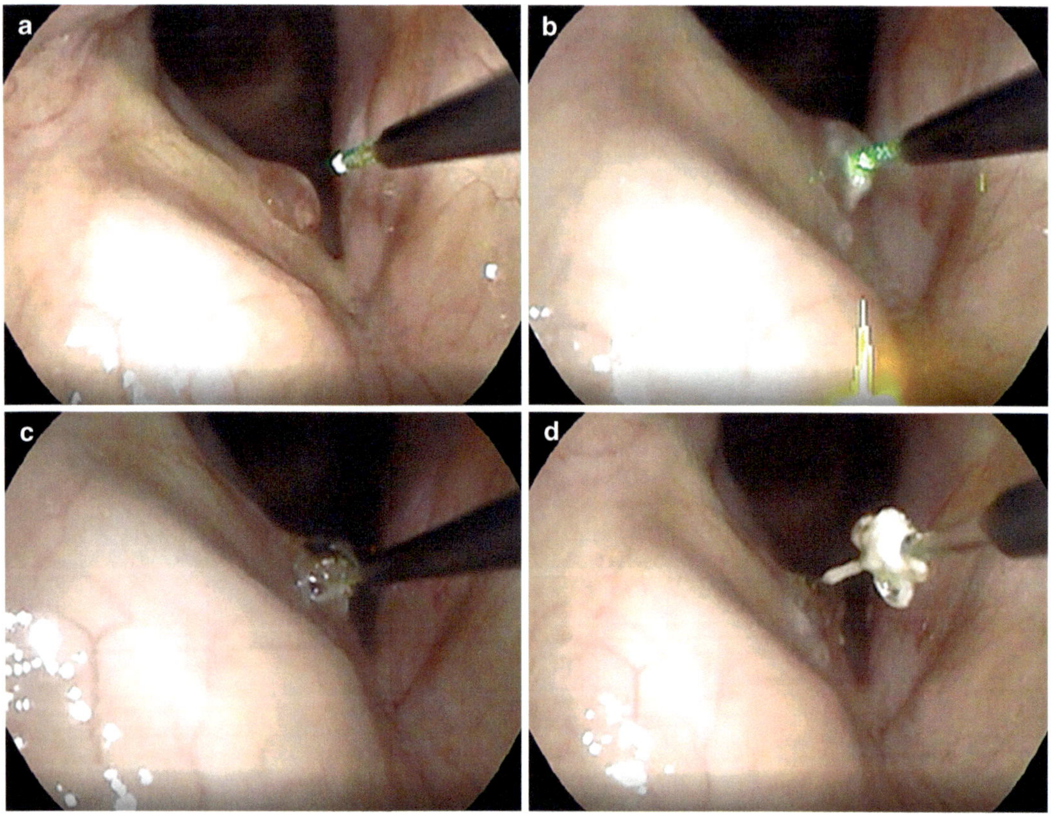

Fig. 3.10 (**a**) An endoscopic view of the larynx prior to surgery showing right hemorrhagic vocal fold polyp. (**b**) A view of the larynx during surgery showing the blue laser glass fiber in contact with the lesion. Note the aberrant strike on the upper surface of the vocal fold anteriorly. (**c**) An endoscopic view of the larynx toward the end of surgery. (**d**) An endoscopic view of the larynx showing how the blue laser glass fiber is used to remove the surgical debris

Fig. 3.11 (**a**) An endoscopic view of the larynx showing a left vocal fold hemorrhagic polyp. Note the reactive lesion on the right vocal fold. (**b**) An endoscopic view of the larynx showing the blue laser in noncontact mode. Note blanching of the lesion. (**c**) An endoscopic view of the larynx showing complete blanching of the polyp following blue laser therapy. (**d**) An endoscopic view showing the blue laser glass fiber coagulating the base of the lesion. (**e**) An endoscopic view showing how the blue laser glass fiber is used to peel off the polyp from the free edge of the left vocal fold. (**f**) An endoscopic view of the larynx showing how the lesion has been removed. (**g**) An endoscopic view of the larynx showing how the cup forceps is used to remove the remaining surgical debris. (**h**) An endoscopic view of the larynx showing injection of dexamethasone into the surgical bed

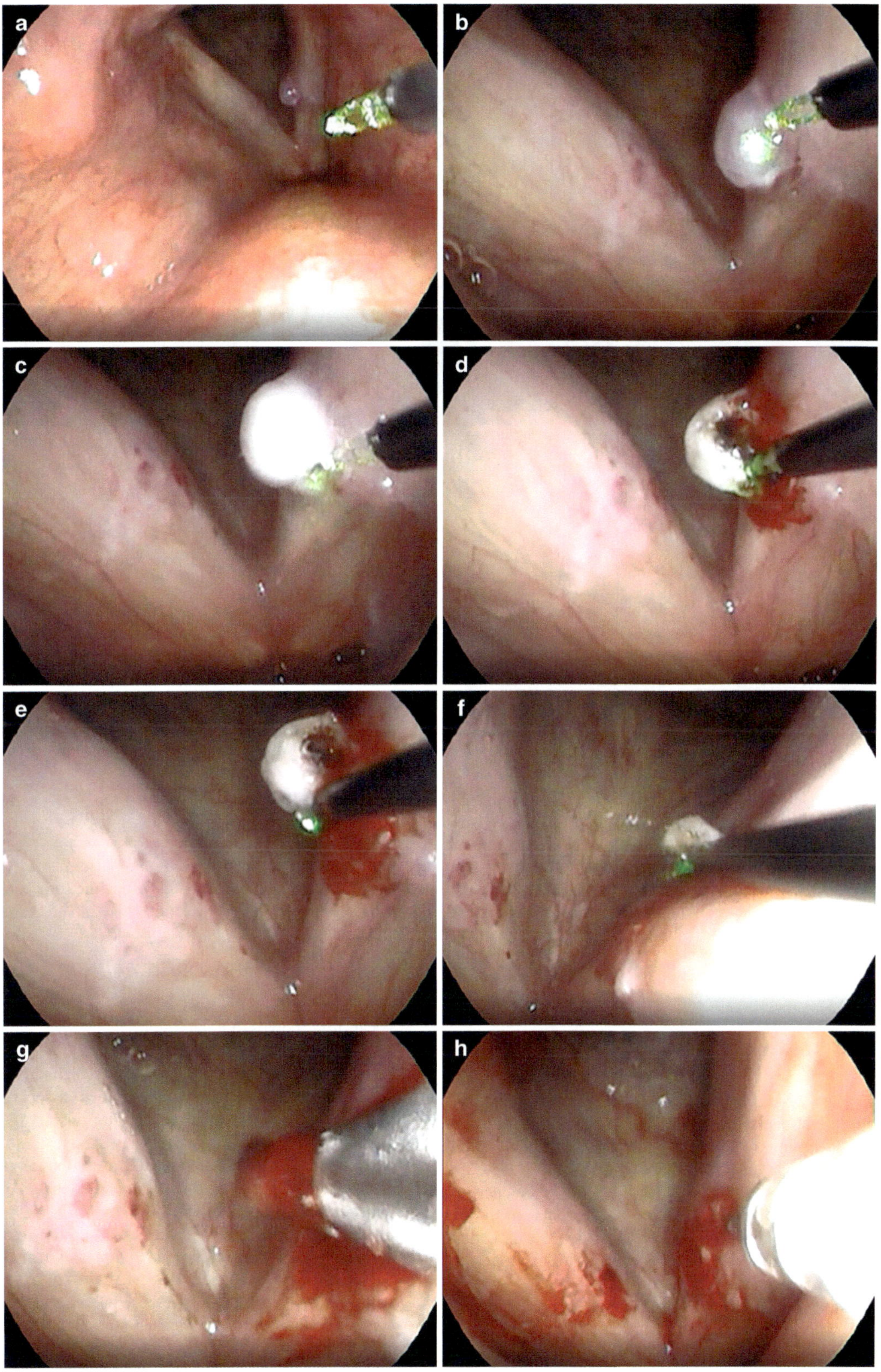
a
b
c
d
e
f
g
h

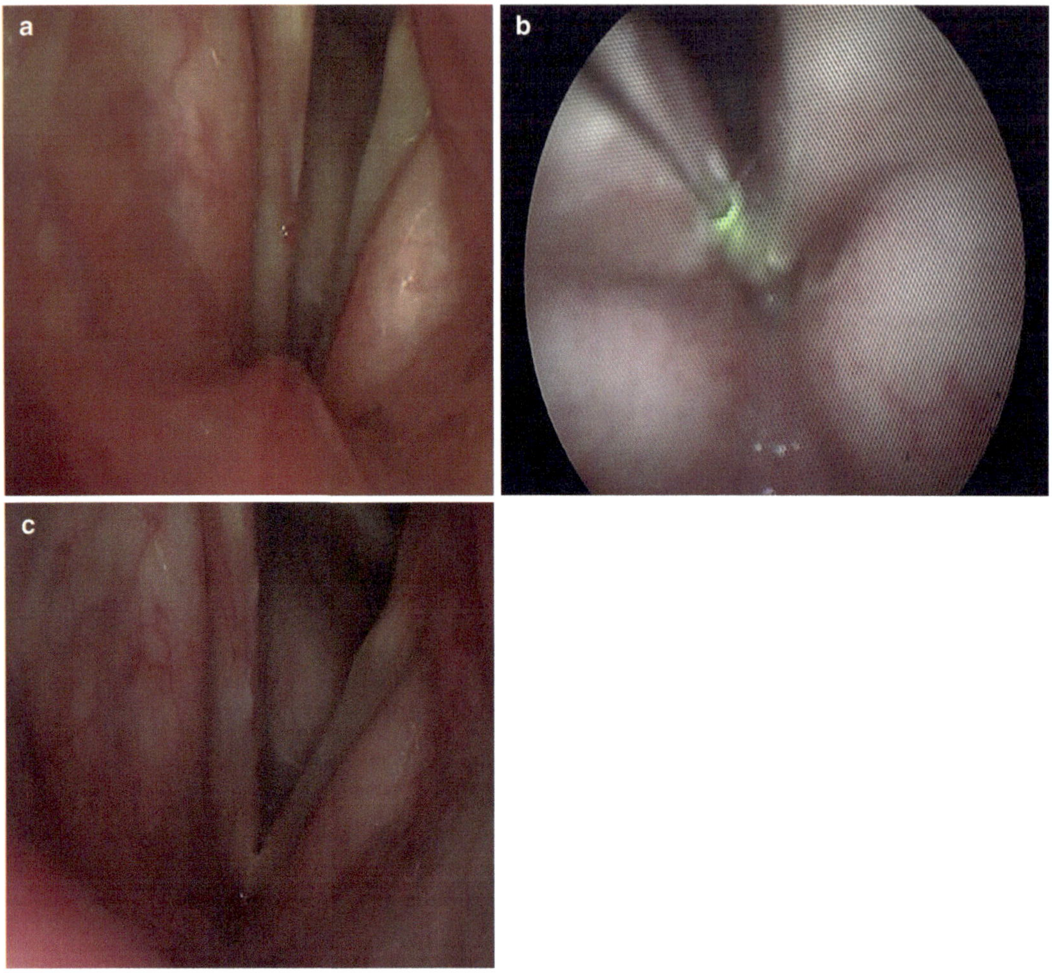

Fig. 3.12 (**a**) Laryngeal examination showing right vocal fold mass with a small adjacent area of leukoplakia. (**b**) In-office blue laser vaporization of right vocal fold mass in contact and noncontact modes. Settings were 6 watts, 40 ms pulse duration, and 300 ms pulse pause. (**c**) Laryngeal examination 6 months after the procedure showing complete mass resection and no recurrent leukoplakia

References

1. Filho JM, Carvalho B, Mizoguchi FM, et al. Characteristics of polypoid lesions in patients undergoing microsurgery of the larynx. Int Arch Otorhinolaryngol. 2013;17(3):279–84.
2. Woo SH, Kim RB, Choi SH, et al. Prevalence of laryngeal disease in South Korea: data from the Korea National Health and Nutrition Examination Survey from 2008 to 2011. Yonsei Med J. 2014;55(2):499–507.
3. Wang L, Tan JJ, Wu T, et al. Association between laryngeal pepsin levels and the presence of vocal fold polyps. Otolaryngol Head Neck Surg. 2017;156(1):144–51.
4. Eckley CA, Swensson J, Duprat Ade C, et al. Incidence of structural vocal fold abnormalities associated with vocal fold polyps. Braz J Otorhinolaryngol. 2008;74(4):508–11.
5. Courey MS, Gardner GM, Stone RE, et al. Endoscopic vocal fold microflap: a three-year experience. Ann Otol Rhinol Laryngol. 1995;104(4 Pt 1):267–73.
6. Sataloff RT, Spiegel JR, Heuer RJ, et al. Laryngeal mini-microflap: a new technique and reassessment of the microflap saga. J Voice. 1995;9(2):198–204.
7. Zeitels SM, Burns JA. Office-based laryngeal laser surgery with the 532-nm pulsed-potassium-titanyl-

phosphate laser. Curr Opin Otolaryngol Head Neck Surg. 2007;15(6):394–400.
8. Koufman JA, Rees CJ, Frazier WD, et al. Office-based laryngeal laser surgery: a review of 443 cases using three wavelengths. Otolaryngol Head Neck Surg. 2007;137(1):146–51.
9. Hamdan AL, Hosri J, Feghali PAR, et al. Office-based blue laser therapy of vocal fold polyps: a cohort of 18 patients: blue laser therapy of vocal fold polyps. Laryngoscope. 2023;133(10):2712–8.
10. Abi Zeid Daou C, Ghanem A, Hosri J, Abou Raji Feghali P, Hamdan AL. Office-based laser therapy in vocal fold polyps: a systematic review and meta-analysis. J Voice. 2023;30:S0892-1997(23)00095-4.

4 Office-Based Blue Laser Therapy for Vocal Fold Reinke's Edema

4.1 Introduction

Reinke's edema (RE) is a benign disease of the vocal folds characterized by excess deposition of gelatinous material in the superficial layer of the lamina propria. Other terms used to describe this disease entity are polypoid corditis, polypoid degeneration, and hypertrophic laryngitis [1, 2]. The main risk factors for RE are smoking and gastroesophageal reflux disease [3, 4], although hypothyroidism and voice abuse may contribute to the development of RE. Women are affected more than men with the main symptoms being deepening of the voice referred to as androphonia, voice fatigue, and inability to project the voice. In severe cases, patients also may complain of shortness of breath and stridor [4, 5]. Phonomicrosurgery using the microflap technique is the treatment of choice for symptomatic patients [6]. Other treatment options include office-based intralesional injection of pharmaceutical agents such as hyaluronidase [7] or steroids [8]. Office-based laser therapy also is effective in the management of RE and has shown promising results [9–12]. This chapter presents cases of RE treated in-office using the blue laser.

Supplementary Information The online version contains supplementary material available at https://doi.org/10.1007/978-3-031-71825-0_4.

4.2 Case Presentations

4.2.1 Case 4.1

A 61-year-old female, heavy smoker, presented to the Voice Clinic (ALH) with hoarseness of a few months' duration associated with globus sensation, throat clearing, and choking. The patient denied any history of voice abuse, allergy, or diagnosed reflux disease. Her Voice Handicap Index-10 (VHI-10) score was 13. Her Dyspnea Severity Index (DSI) was 11. Acoustic analysis showed a fundamental frequency (F0) of 128.73 Hz, a habitual pitch (HP) of 129.18 Hz, jitter 2.26, shimmer 7.53, noise-to-harmonic ratio (NHR) of 0.28, and voice turbulence index (VTI) of 0.031. Aerodynamic analysis showed a maximum phonation time (MPT) of 5.02 seconds. Laryngeal flexible endoscopic evaluation revealed bilateral Reinke's edema (RE), type 3 on the right and type 1 on the left using the Tan et al. classification [1]. The patient underwent office-based blue laser therapy for her left vocal fold RE using contact and noncontact modes (Fig. 4.1a and b; Video 4.1). The setting was as follows: power 10 watts, pulse duration 40 ms, and pulse pause time 300 ms. A total of 104 Joules was delivered. Following laser therapy, 0.1 ml of dexamethasone (8 mg/2 ml) was injected into the left vocal fold using a 25-gauge flexible needle that was introduced through the working channel of the endoscope. The procedure was tolerated

A. L. Hamdan et al., *Atlas of Office-based Blue Laser Therapy in Laryngology*,
https://doi.org/10.1007/978-3-031-71825-0_4

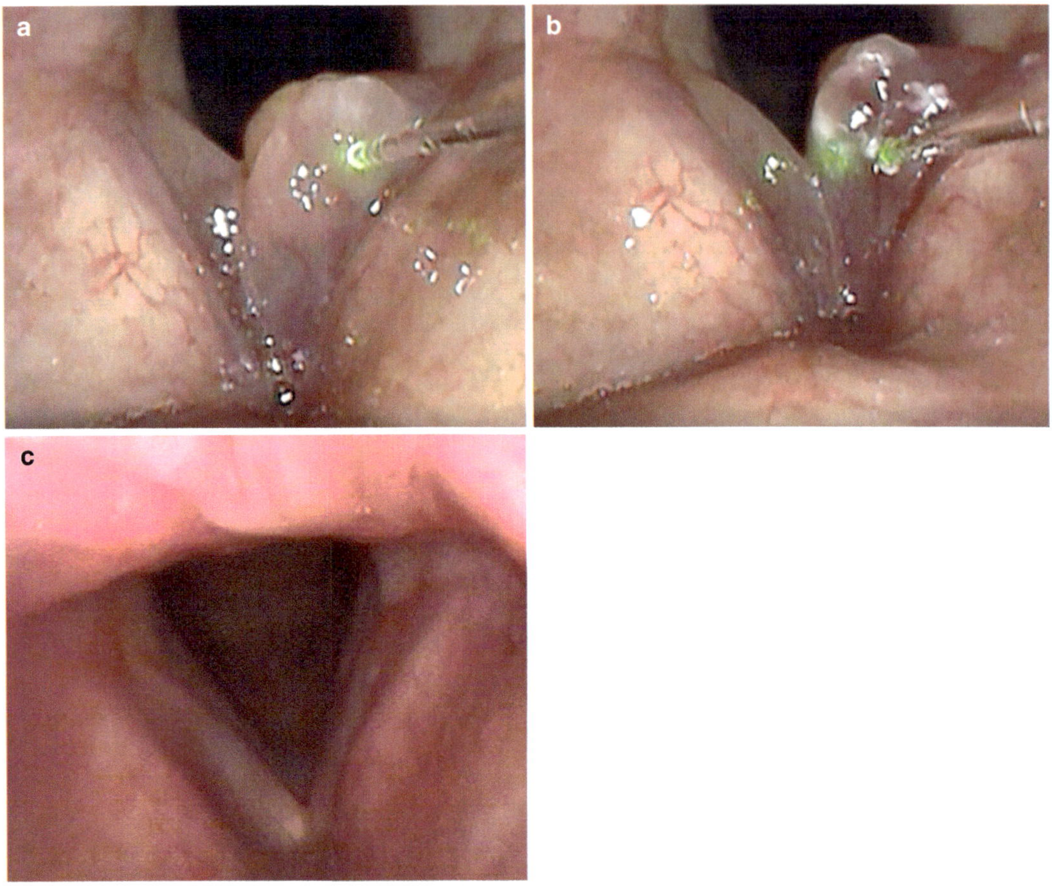

Fig. 4.1 (**a**) An endoscopic view of the larynx showing the blue laser glass fiber (400 micrometer) in near-contact with the left vocal fold. Note blanching of the lesion at the site of the laser. (**b**) An endoscopic view of the larynx showing the blue laser glass fiber (400 micrometer) in contact with the lesion. (**c**) A view of the larynx 6 weeks after surgery showing almost complete regression of the lesion on the left side. Note mild residual edema and redness at the surgical site

well by the patient with no complications noted. On follow-up 6 weeks later, the patient had significant improvement in her voice quality. Her VHI-10 score dropped to 0. Her DSI dropped to 2. Acoustic analysis showed an increase in the F0 to 167.7 Hz, and an increase in the HP to 154.74 Hz. There was a decrease in jitter to 0.35 and in shimmer to 1.16. Her MPT increased to 18.07 seconds. Laryngeal examination revealed almost complete regression of the RE of the left vocal fold except for mild edema and redness at the surgical bed (Fig. 4.1c).

4.2.2 Case 4.2

A 60-year-old female, heavy smoker, presented to the Voice Clinic (ALH) with voice fatigue and deepening of her voice of a few years' duration. Her voice symptoms were associated with aspiration, odynophonia, and mild dyspnea. The patient had a history of reflux disease and denied any history of allergy or voice abuse. Her Voice Handicap Index-10 (VHI-10) score was 19. Her Dyspnea Severity Index (DSI) was 8. Acoustic analysis showed a fundamental frequency (F0) of 89.5 Hz, habitual pitch (HP) of 100.41 Hz, jitter 2.43, shimmer 9.27, noise-to-harmonic ratio (NHR) of 0.2, and voice turbulence index (VTI) of 0.135. Aerodynamic analysis showed a maximum phonation time (MPT) of 5 seconds. Laryngeal examination revealed type 3 Reinke's edema (RE) of the left vocal fold and type 2 of the right vocal fold (Fig. 4.2a).

The patient underwent office-based blue laser therapy for her bilateral RE using contact and noncontact modes (Fig. 4.2b–e; Video 4.2). The procedure was tolerated well by the patient with no complications noted.

On follow-up 6 weeks after surgery, the patient had marked improvement in her voice quality and in her breathing. Her VHI-10 score dropped to 2, and her DSI dropped to 1. Acoustic analysis showed an increase in the F0 to 182.5 Hz and in the HP to 142.5 Hz. There was a decrease in shimmer to 2.42. Laryngeal examination revealed almost complete disease regression bilaterally (Fig. 4.2f).

4.2.3 Case 4.3

A 57-year-old male, heavy smoker, presented to the Voice Clinic (ALH) with hoarseness of a few months' duration. The patient denied any history of phonotrauma, allergy, or reflux disease. Her Voice Handicap Index-10 (VHI-10) score at presentation was 30. Acoustic analysis showed a fundamental frequency (F0) of 207.2 Hz, jitter 2.35, shimmer 5.19, noise-to-harmonics ratio (NHR) of 0.15, and voice turbulence index (VTI) of 0.04. Aerodynamic analysis showed a maximum phonation time (MPT) of 10.16 seconds. Laryngeal examination revealed bilateral type 1 Reinke's edema (RE) of the vocal folds (Fig. 4.3a). The patient underwent office-based blue laser therapy using mostly the noncontact mode. The laser setting was as follows: Power 10 watts, pulse duration 40 ms, and pulse pause 300 ms (Fig. 4.3b; Video 4.3). On follow-up 6 weeks later, the patient had marked improvement in her voice quality. Her VHI-10 score dropped to 1. Acoustic analysis showed a decrease in jitter to 0.84 and in shimmer to 2.36. Aerodynamic analysis showed an increase in her MPT to 16.82. Laryngeal examination revealed almost complete regression of the RE bilaterally.

4.2.4 Case 4.4

A 61-year-old male, heavy smoker, presented to the Voice Clinic (ALH) with a history of hoarseness that had been worsening over the last few years. The patient had history of voice abuse but denied any history of allergy or reflux disease. His Voice Handicap Index-10 (VHI-10) score was 20. His Dyspnea Severity Index (DSI) was 8. Laryngeal flexible endoscopic examination revealed bilateral type 3 Reinke's edema (RE). The patient underwent office-based blue laser therapy for his bilateral RE (Fig. 4.4a; Video 4.4). Following laser therapy, 0.2 ml of dexamethasone (8 mg/2 ml) was injected into each vocal fold. The procedure was well tolerated by the patient. On follow-up 6 weeks after surgery, the patient had substantial improvement in his voice quality. His VHI-10 score dropped to 0, and his DSI dropped to 4. Laryngeal examination revealed almost complete regression of the lesion bilaterally with mild residual inflammation and whitish discoloration at the free edge of the vocal folds (Fig. 4.4b). It is important to note that the patient did not rest his voice after surgery and did not stop smoking.

4.2.5 Case 4.5

A 67-year-old female, heavy smoker, presented to the Voice Clinic (ALH) with hoarseness of a few years' duration. The patient denied any history of voice abuse, allergy or reflux disease. Her Voice Handicap Index-10 (VHI-10) score was 12. Her Dyspnea Severity Index (DSI) was 7. Acoustic analysis showed a fundamental frequency (F0) of 91.92 Hz, jitter 1.26, shimmer 5.7, noise-to-harmonics ratio (NHR) of 0.18, and

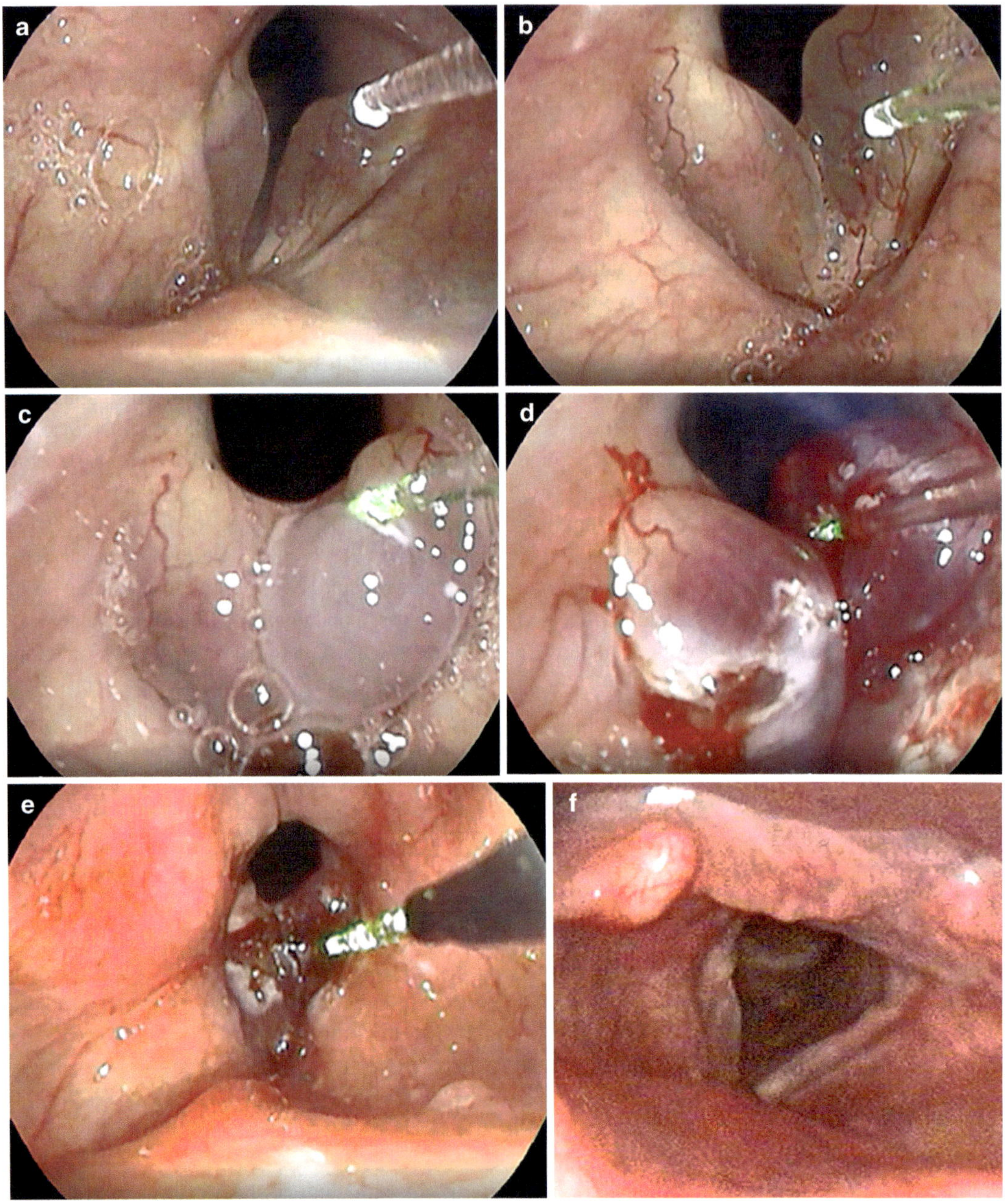

Fig. 4.2 (**a**) A view of the larynx showing type 3 Reinke's edema (RE) of the left vocal fold and type 2 of the right vocal fold. (**b**) Intraoperative view of the larynx showing the laser glass fiber approaching the lesion on the left side. (**c**) An intraoperative view showing the blue laser in contact mode against the RE of the left vocal fold. (**d**) View of the larynx half-way through surgery. (**e**) Intraoperative view toward the end of surgery showing blanching of the lesion of the right vocal fold with disruption of the mucosal lining. (**f**) Postoperative view 6 weeks later showing complete disease regression on the left side and partial disease regression on the right side

voice turbulence index (VTI) of 0.067. Aerodynamic analysis showed a maximum phonation time (MPT) of 4 seconds. Laryngeal examination revealed bilateral type 3 Reinke's edema (RE) of the vocal folds. The patient underwent office-based blue laser therapy for her vocal

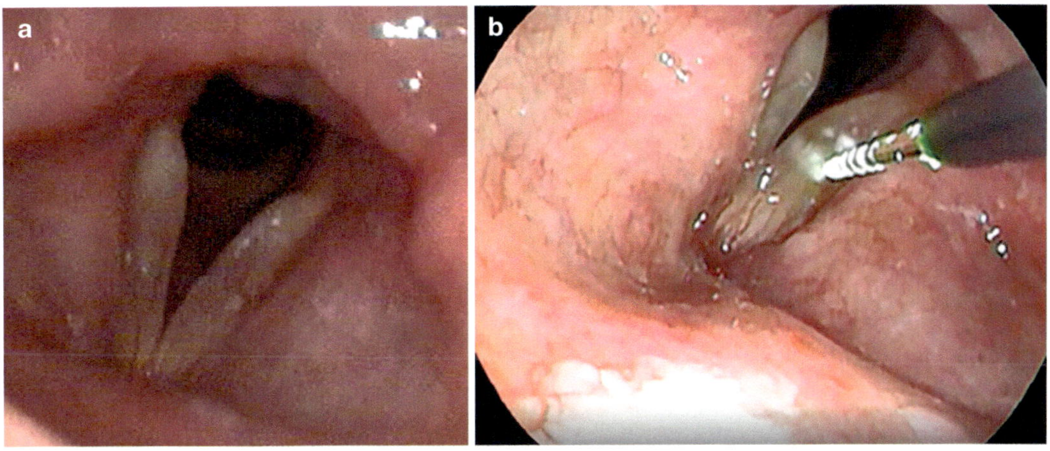

Fig. 4.3 (**a**) Preoperative view of the larynx showing type 1 Reinke's edema of both vocal folds. (**b**) Intraoperative view showing the blue laser glass fiber in noncontact mode

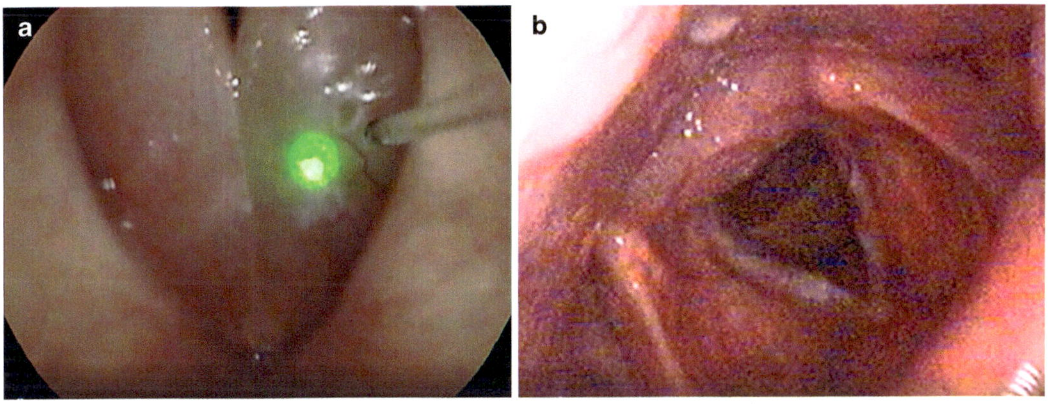

Fig. 4.4 (**a**) Intraoperative view of the vocal folds showing the blue laser beam aiming at the Reinke's edema of the left vocal fold (**b**) A postoperative view of the larynx six weeks following surgery showing partial regression of the Reinke's edema bilaterally. Note blanching and mild edema on the free edge of the vocal folds

fold RE using contact and noncontact modes (Fig. 4.5a–c; Video 4.5). The procedure was tolerated well by the patient with no complications noted. The patient was lost for follow up for 2 years, following which she presented to the Voice Clinic with mild dysphonia but marked improvement in her voice quality in comparison to her first presentation. Her VHI-10 score dropped to 1 and her DSI dropped to 3. Acoustic analysis showed an increase in F0 to 148.67 Hz, and a decrease in shimmer to 2.79. Aerodynamic analysis revealed an increase in her MPT to 19.15 seconds. Laryngeal examination showed type 2 RE of the right vocal fold and type 1 RE of the left vocal fold (Fig. 4.5d). The patient elected to undergo another session of office-based blue laser with intralesional steroid injection (0.1 ml of dexamethasone 8 mg/2 ml). The procedure was tolerated well by the patient with no complications noted.

4.2.6 Case 4.6

A 61-year-old female presented to the Voice Clinic (ALH) with progressive hoarseness of a few years' duration. The patient had no symptoms related to breathing or swallowing, and she

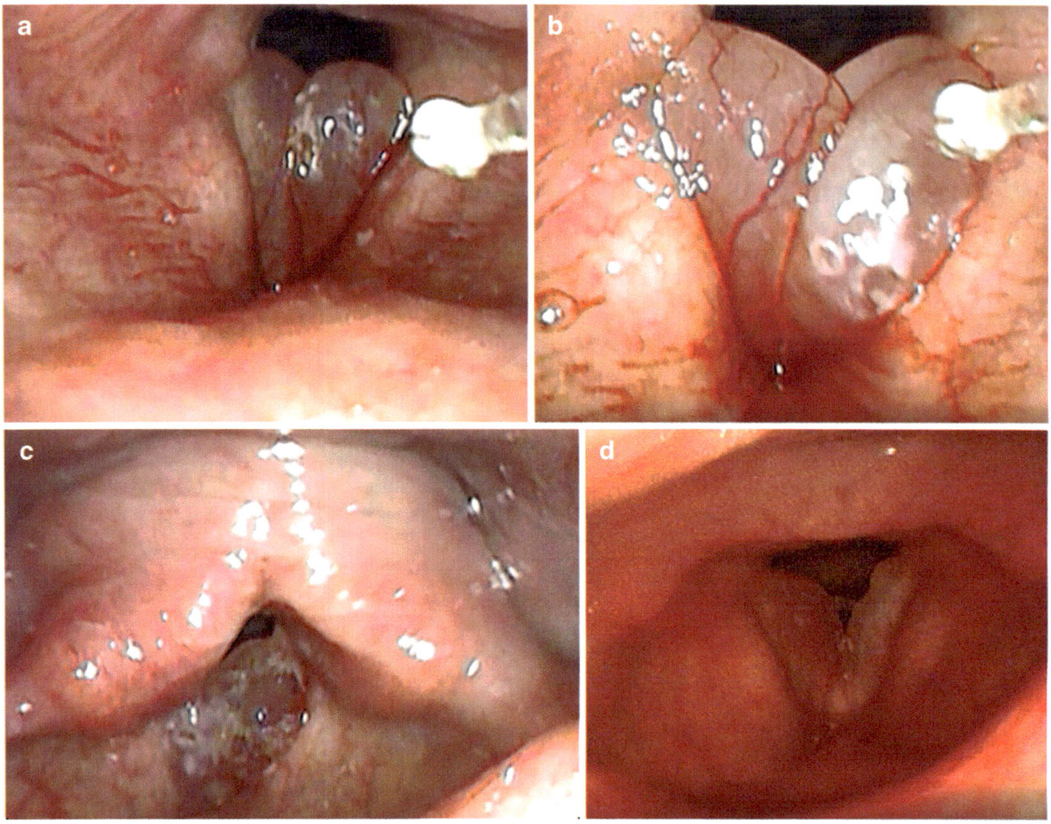

Fig. 4.5 (**a**) An intraoperative view of the larynx showing the extent of the Reinke's edema (RE) which was narrowing 70–80% of the airway. (**b**) Another intraoperative view showing blanching of the RE on the left side following application of the blue laser in noncontact mode. (**c**) An image of the vocal folds toward the end of the blue laser therapy session. (**d**) Postoperative view of the larynx 2 years after surgery showing partial disease regression (type 1 RE) of the left vocal fold and type 2 RE of the right vocal fold with hyperemia and dilated vessels on the upper surface

denied any history of reflux disease or allergy. The patient had a history of voice overuse/abuse and heavy smoking. Her Voice Handicap Index −10 (VHI-10) score on presentation was 20. Acoustic analysis showed a fundamental frequency (F_0) of 114.93 Hz, habitual pitch (HP) of 112.3 Hz, jitter 1.44, shimmer 6.14, noise-to-harmonic ratio (NHR) of 0.154, and voice turbulence index (VTI) of 0.048. Her maximum phonation time (MPT) was 2.34 seconds. On laryngeal examination, she had type 1 Reinke's edema (RE) on the left vocal fold and type 3 RE on the right vocal fold. Careful examination also showed leukoplakia on the upper lip of the left vocal fold (Fig. 4.6a). The patient underwent office-based biopsy of the left vocal fold lesion (Fig. 4.6b). The vocal fold biopsy was followed by blue laser therapy for her RE (Fig. 4.6c). The laser setting used was power 10 watts, pulse duration 40 ms, and pulse pause 300 ms. A total of 120 J was given during the procedure. The laser was used in contact and noncontact modes. Histopathologic examination of the left vocal fold lesion showed high-grade dysplasia. The patient underwent another office-based blue laser therapy for her left vocal fold lesion. Laser was used at a power of 10 watts, pulse duration 30 ms, and pulse pause 300 ms. A total of 56 Joules was given during the procedure. Six weeks after the second surgery, the patient presented with marked improvement in her voice quality. Her VHI-10 score was 5. Acoustic analysis postoperatively

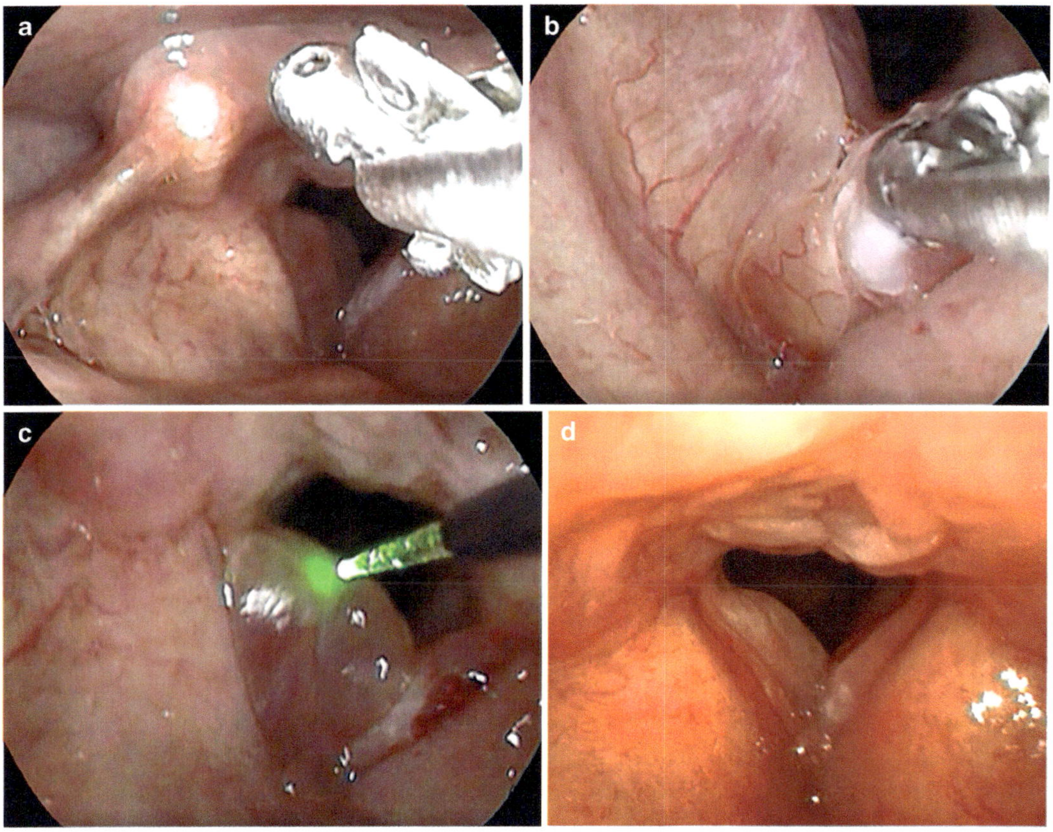

Fig. 4.6 (**a**) An endoscopic view of the larynx showing the cup forceps targeting the left vocal fold lesion. (**b**) An endoscopic view of the larynx showing the biopsy of the left vocal fold lesion. (**c**) An intraoperative view showing blanching of the right vocal fold Reinke's edema (RE) following the application of the blue laser in noncontact mode. (**d**) An endoscopic view of the larynx eight weeks following surgery showing type 1 RE of the left vocal fold and partial regression of the RE of the right vocal fold

showed an F_0 of 152.93 Hz, HP of 135.6 Hz, jitter of 0.77, shimmer of 2.95, NHR of 0.138, and VTI of 0.040. Her MPT was 4.28 seconds. Laryngeal endoscopic examination showed partial regression of RE of the right vocal fold, and partial regression of the left vocal fold lesion (Fig. 4.6d). The patient was satisfied with the result and elected not to undergo further treatment.

4.2.7 Case 4.7

A 76 year-old-female, heavy smoker, presented to the Voice Clinic (ALH) with hoarseness of few years duration. The patient denied any history of phonotrauma, allergy, or reflux disease. Her Voice Handicap Index-10 (VHI-10) score was 7. Acoustic analysis showed a fundamental frequency (F0) of 104 Hz, habitual pitch (HP) of 125 Hz, jitter 5, shimmer 1.73, noise-to-harmonic ratio (NHR) of 0.45, and voice turbulence index (VTI) of 0.123. Her maximum phonation time (MPT) was 10.65 seconds. Laryngeal flexible examination revealed type 1 Reinke's edema (RE) of the right vocal fold and type 3 RE of the left vocal fold. The patient underwent office-based blue laser therapy for bilateral RE using contact and noncontact modes. A total of 189 Joules was delivered. The procedure was tolerated well by the patient with no complications noted (Fig. 4.7a; Video 4.6). On follow-up 6 weeks later, the patient had marked improve-

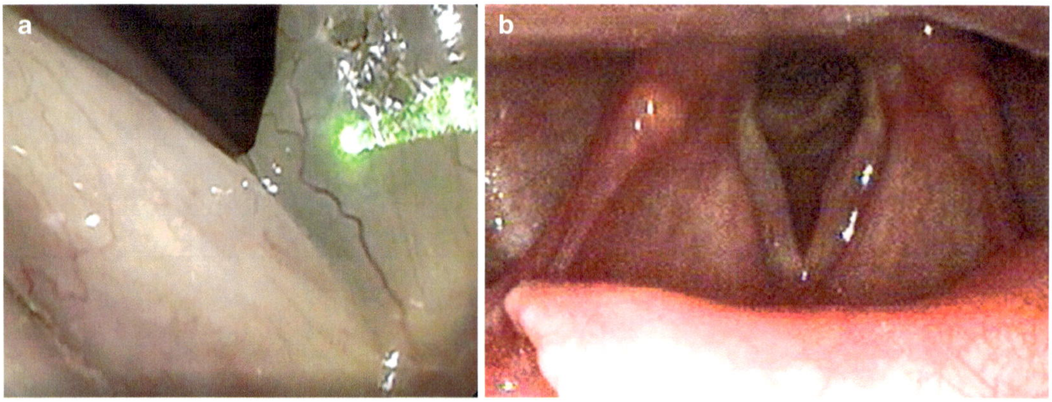

Fig. 4.7 (**a**) An intraoperative view of the larynx showing the blue laser beam aiming at the left vocal fold Reinke's edema (RE). (**b**) Laryngeal examination 7 weeks after surgery showing complete disease regression of the right vocal fold RE and partial disease regression of the left vocal fold RE

ment in her voice quality. Her VHI-10 score dropped to 1. Postoperative acoustic analysis revealed an increase in the F0 to 134.23 Hz. There was a decrease in jitter to 2.6, shimmer to 1.5, NHR to 0.3 and VTI to 0.06. Laryngeal examination revealed complete disease regression of the RE of the right vocal fold and partial disease regression of the RE of the left vocal fold (Fig. 4.7b). The patient elected to undergo a second office-based blue laser therapy for her residual edema of the left vocal fold. The procedure was tolerated well by the patient with no complications noted.

4.2.8 Case 4.8

A 44-year-old woman presented to the Voice Clinic (ALH) with hoarseness that had been worsening over the last few years. The patient had history of phonotrauma and denied any history of smoking, allergy, or reflux disease. Her Voice Handicap Index-10 (VHI-10) score was 22. Acoustic analysis showed a showed a fundamental frequency (F0) of 227 Hz, habitual pitch (HP) of 209.41 Hz, jitter 2, shimmer 8.25, noise-to-harmonic ratio (NHR) of 0.154, and voice turbulence index (VTI) of 0.045. Her maximum phonation time (MPT) was 8.82 seconds. Laryngeal examination revealed bilateral type 2 Reinke's edema (RE) (Fig. 4.8a).

The patient underwent office-based blue laser therapy for the bilateral RE using contact and noncontact modes. A total of 25 Joules was delivered to the right vocal fold, and 22.8 Joules was delivered to the left vocal fold (Fig. 4.8b). Following the laser therapy, 0.2 ml of dexamethasone (8 mg/2 ml) was injected into both vocal folds using the 25-gauge flexible needle via the transnasal approach. The procedure was tolerated well by the patient with no complications noted. On follow-up 6 weeks later, the patient had marked improvement in her voice quality. Her VHI-10 score dropped to 1. Postoperative acoustic analysis showed an increase in the F0 to 242.15 Hz, in HP to 240.71. There was a decrease in jitter to 0.515 and in shimmer to 2.55. There was an increase in her MPT to 20.9 seconds. Laryngeal examination revealed almost complete regression of the lesions (Fig. 4.8c). The patient was advised to follow-up in 6 weeks for a possible office-based steroid injection.

4.2.9 Case 4.9

A 54-year-old woman presented to the Voice Clinic (ALH) with a history of hoarseness of a few months duration. The patient had a history of smoking and voice abuse but denied any history of reflux disease or allergy. Her Voice Handicap Index-10 (VHI-10) score on presentation was 17.

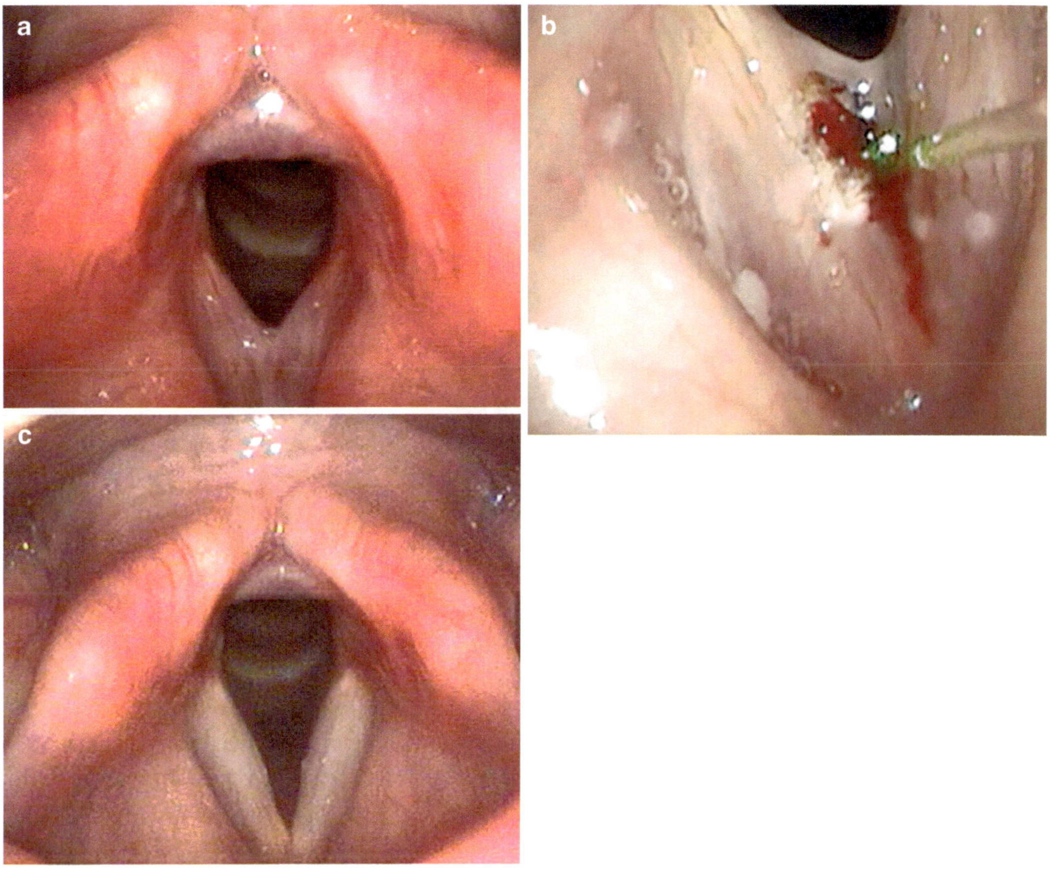

Fig. 4.8 (**a**) An endoscopic view of the larynx showing type 2 Reinke's edema of both vocal folds. Note that the vocal folds are in contact during inhalation. (**b**) An intraoperative view showing blanching of the right vocal fold with incision of the mucosal cover on the upper surface. (**c**) A postoperative view of the larynx 6 weeks following surgery showing almost complete disease regression bilaterally. Note the mucosal irregularity on the free edge of the vocal fold

Acoustic analysis showed a fundamental frequency (F0) of 129.3 Hz, habitual pitch (HP) of 133.4 Hz, jitter 5.59, shimmer 17.51, noise-to-harmonic ratio (NHR) of 0.268, and voice turbulence index (VTI) of 0.052. Her maximum phonation time (MPT) was 4.3 seconds. On laryngeal examination, she had bilateral type 1 Reinke's edema (RE). The patient underwent office-based blue laser therapy for both vocal folds under local anesthesia using a power of 10 watts, pulse duration 40 ms, and pulse pause 300 ms. A total of 126 Joules was given during the procedure (Fig. 4.9a). Six weeks after the surgery, the patient presented with marked improvement in her voice quality. Acoustic analysis showed a F_0 of 141.1 Hz, HP of 140.8 Hz, jitter of 1.56, shimmer of 3.41, NHR of 0.148, and VTI of 0.04. Her MPT was 8.14 seconds. Laryngeal examination showed partial regression of RE, left more than right (Fig. 4.9b).

4.2.10 Case 4.10

A 53-year-old woman presented to the Voice Clinic (ALH) with a long history of hoarseness associated with dyspnea and difficulty breathing. The patient was a smoker but denied any history of phonotrauma, reflux disease, or allergy. Her Voice Handicap Index-10 (VHI-10) score on pre-

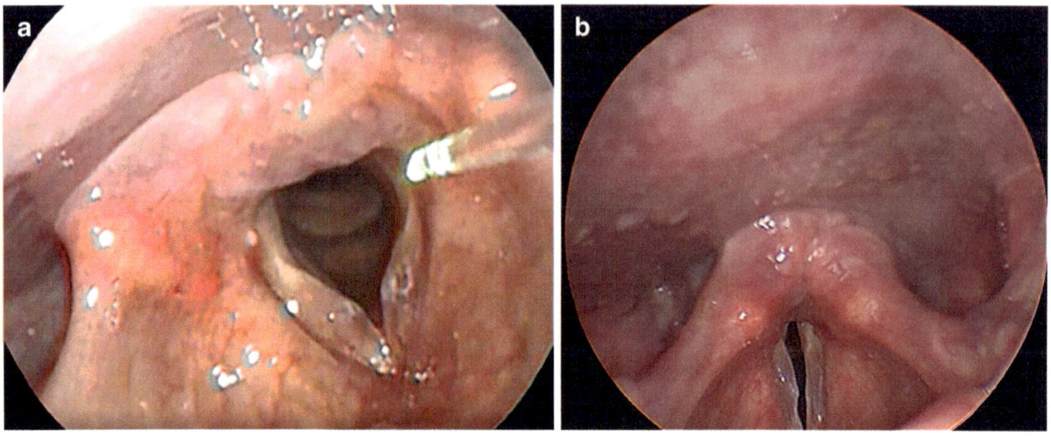

Fig. 4.9 (**a**) Intraoperative view of the vocal folds during office-based blue laser therapy. Note blanching of vocal folds. (**b**) A video-stroboscopic examination of the larynx six weeks after surgery showing improvement in the Reinke's edema on the left side and mild residual disease on the right. There was no impairment in the mucosal waves following treatment

sentation was 18. The Dyspnea Severity Index (DSI) and the STOP-BANG (for obstructive sleep apnea) scores were 33 and 4, respectively. Acoustic analysis showed a fundamental frequency (F_0) of 108.9 Hz, habitual pitch (HP) of 94.7 Hz, jitter 0.35, shimmer 2.39, noise-to-harmonic ratio (NHR) of 0.137, and voice turbulence index (VTI) of 0.037. Her maximum phonation time (MPT) was 3.59 seconds. On laryngeal examination, she had bilateral type 3 Reinke's edema (RE). The patient underwent office-based blue laser therapy under local anesthesia using a power of 10 watts, pulse duration 40 ms, and pulse pause 300 ms. A total of 112 Joules was given (Fig. 4.10a; Video 4.7). The laser was used in contact and noncontact modes. Four weeks after the surgery, the patient presented with moderate improvement in her voice quality and a decrease in her VHI-10 score to 2. Acoustic analysis postoperatively showed an F_0 of 162.1 Hz, HP of 120.75 Hz, jitter of 0.33, shimmer of 2.16, NHR of 0.125, and VTI of 0.036. Her MPT was 5.09 seconds. The patient had also marked improvement in her breathing. Her DSI dropped to 6, and her STOP-BANG score dropped to 2. Laryngeal endoscopic exam showed type 1 RE of the right vocal fold and type 2 on the left (Fig. 4.10b).

4.2.11 Case 4.11

A 63-year-old woman presented to the Voice Clinic (ALH) with a history of hoarseness associated with mild dyspnea. The patient was a smoker but denied any history of phonotrauma, reflux disease, or allergy. Her Voice Handicap Index −10 (VHI-10) score on presentation was 30. The Dyspnea Severity Index (DSI) score was 6, and her STOP-BANG score was 5. Acoustic analysis showed a fundamental frequency (F_0) of 110.1 Hz, habitual pitch (HP) of 122.6 Hz, jitter 3.85, shimmer 17.69, noise-to-harmonic ratio (NHR) of 0.272, and voice turbulence index (VTI) of 0.098. Her maximum phonation time (MPT) was 18 seconds. On laryngeal examination, she had bilateral type 3 Reinke's edema (RE) (Fig. 4.11a). The patient underwent office-based blue laser therapy for both vocal folds under local anesthesia using a power of 10 watts, pulse duration 40 ms, and pulse pause 300 ms. She received a total of 273 Joules during the procedure (Fig. 4.11b; Video 4.8). Seven weeks after the surgery, the patient presented with marked improvement in her voice quality and breathing. Her VHI-10 score dropped to 6, her DSI score dropped to 0, and her STOP-BANG score dropped to 2. Acoustic analysis postoperatively

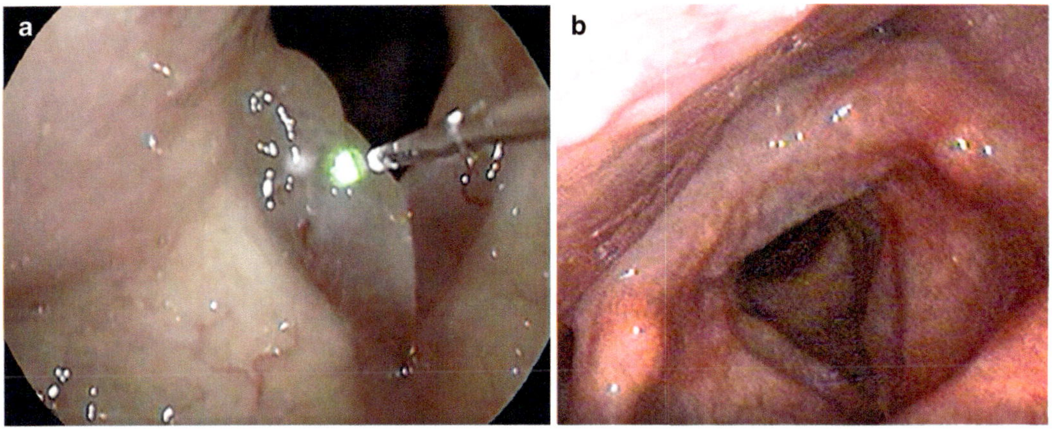

Fig. 4.10 (**a**) Intraoperative view of the larynx showing the blue laser glass fiber in near-contact mode. Note blanching of the Reinke's edema at the site of treatment. (**b**) A postoperative view of the larynx 4 weeks after treatment showing almost complete regression of the disease on the right side and mild improvement on the left. Note the residual edema and hyperemia which is expected to resolve about 6 to 8 weeks after surgery

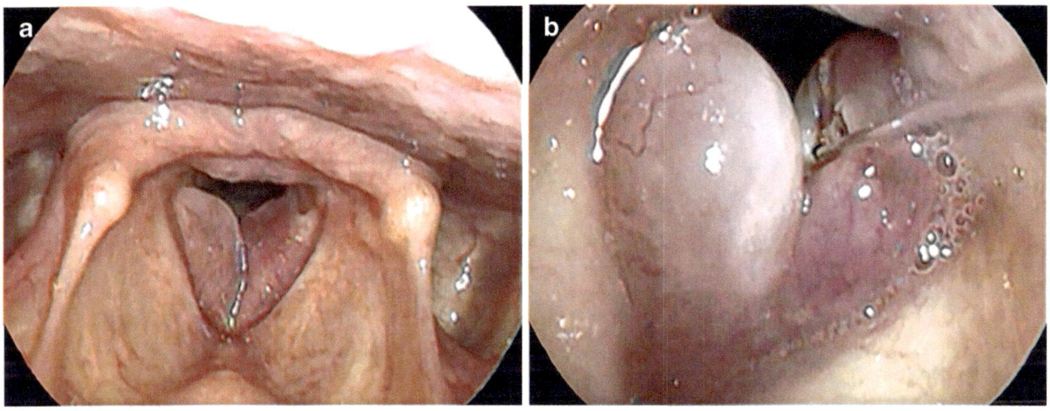

Fig. 4.11 (**a**) Preoperative view of the larynx showing type 3 Reinke's edema bilaterally. (**b**) Intraoperative view of the larynx showing the blue laser glass fiber in contact mode against the left vocal fold Reinke's edema

showed a marked decrease in jitter to 2.99, shimmer to 2.75, NHR to 0.235, and VTI of 0.052. Her MPT was 18.4 seconds. Laryngeal endoscopic examination showed marked reduction in the size of the RE of both vocal folds.

4.2.12 Case 4.12

A 74-year-old male, heavy smoker, presented to the Voice Clinic (ALH) with hoarseness of a few months duration associated with dyspnea and difficulty breathing. The patient had no history of phonotrauma, reflux disease, or allergy. His Voice Handicap Index-10 (VHI-10) score on presentation was 26. The Dyspnea Severity Index (DSI) and STOP-BANG scores were 23 and 5, respectively. On laryngeal examination, he had type 3 Reinke's edema (RE) of the left vocal fold and type 2 on the right. The patient underwent office-based blue laser therapy for both vocal folds under local anesthesia using a power of 10 watts, pulse duration 40 ms, and pulse pause 300 ms. A total of 120 Joules were given during the procedure. The laser was used in contact and noncontact modes and was followed by a steroid injection in the surgical bed (Fig. 4.12a and b; Video 4.9). Five weeks after the surgery, the patient pre-

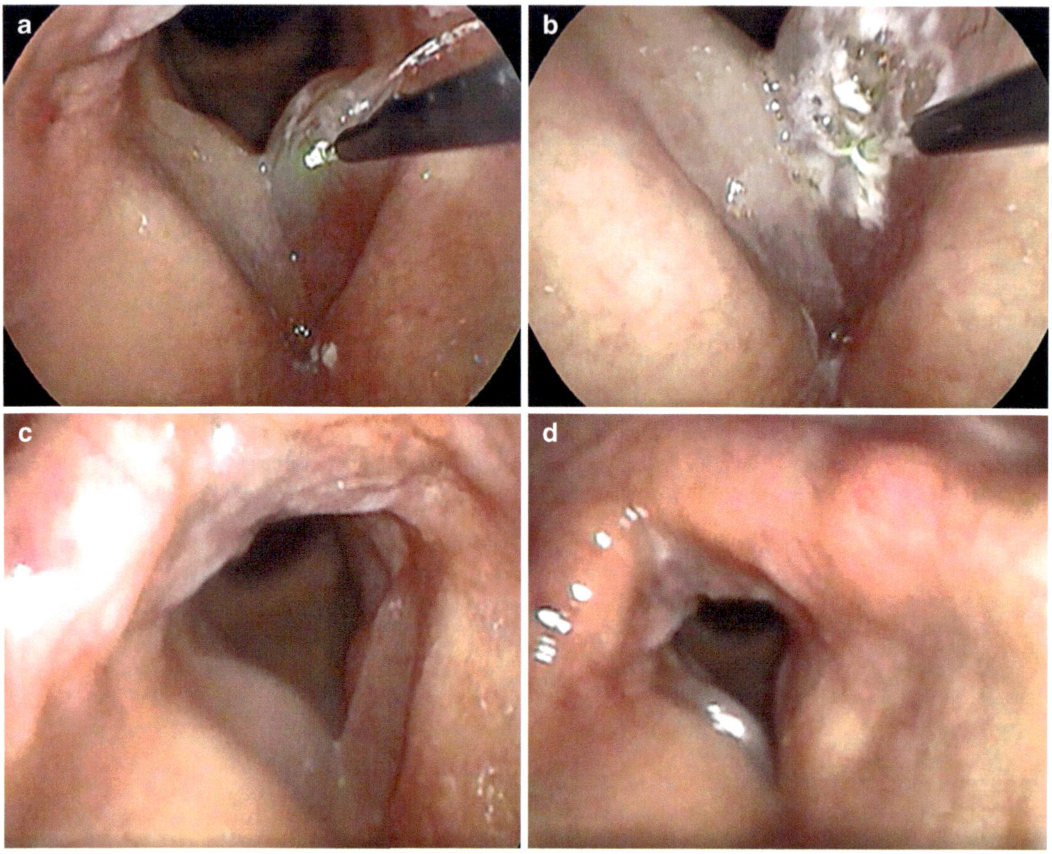

Fig. 4.12 (**a**) Intraoperative view of the larynx showing the blue laser application in noncontact mode. (**b**) Intraoperative view of the larynx showing blue laser application in contact mode. (**c**) View of the larynx six weeks after surgery showing marked regression in the Reinke's edema bilaterally. (**d**) An endoscopic view of the larynx 12 weeks after surgery showing further disease regression and decrease in vocal fold edema

sented with mild improvement in his voice quality but marked improvement in his breathing. His VHI-10 score decreased to 17, his DSI to 6, and his STOP-BANG score to 3. Laryngeal endoscopic examination showed marked disease regression (Fig. 4.12c). Three months later he presented with further improvement in his voice and decrease in his vocal fold edema (Fig. 4.12d).

4.2.13 Case 4.13

A 56-year-old female, heavy smoker, presented to the Voice Clinic (ALH) with hoarseness of a few years duration. The patient had no other symptoms, and her medical history was essentially negative for reflux disease. Her Voice Handicap Index 10 (VHI-10) score was 20, her Dyspnea Severity Index (DSI) score was 12, and her STOP-BANG score was 3. Acoustic analysis showed a fundamental frequency (Fo) of 111.9 Hz, habitual pitch (HP) of 92.5 Hz, and noise-to-harmonic ratio (NHR) of 0.125. On laryngeal examination, she had bilateral type 3 Reinke's edema (RE) (Fig. 4.13a). She underwent office-based blue laser therapy using a power of 10 watts, pulse duration 40 ms, and pause pulse 300 ms (Fig. 4.13b). The procedure was tolerated well by the patient, and no complications were noted. At eight weeks following surgery, the patient had marked improvement in her voice quality and breathing. Her VHI-10 score dropped to 10, her DSI score dropped to 1, and her STOP-BANG score decreased to 2. Acoustic

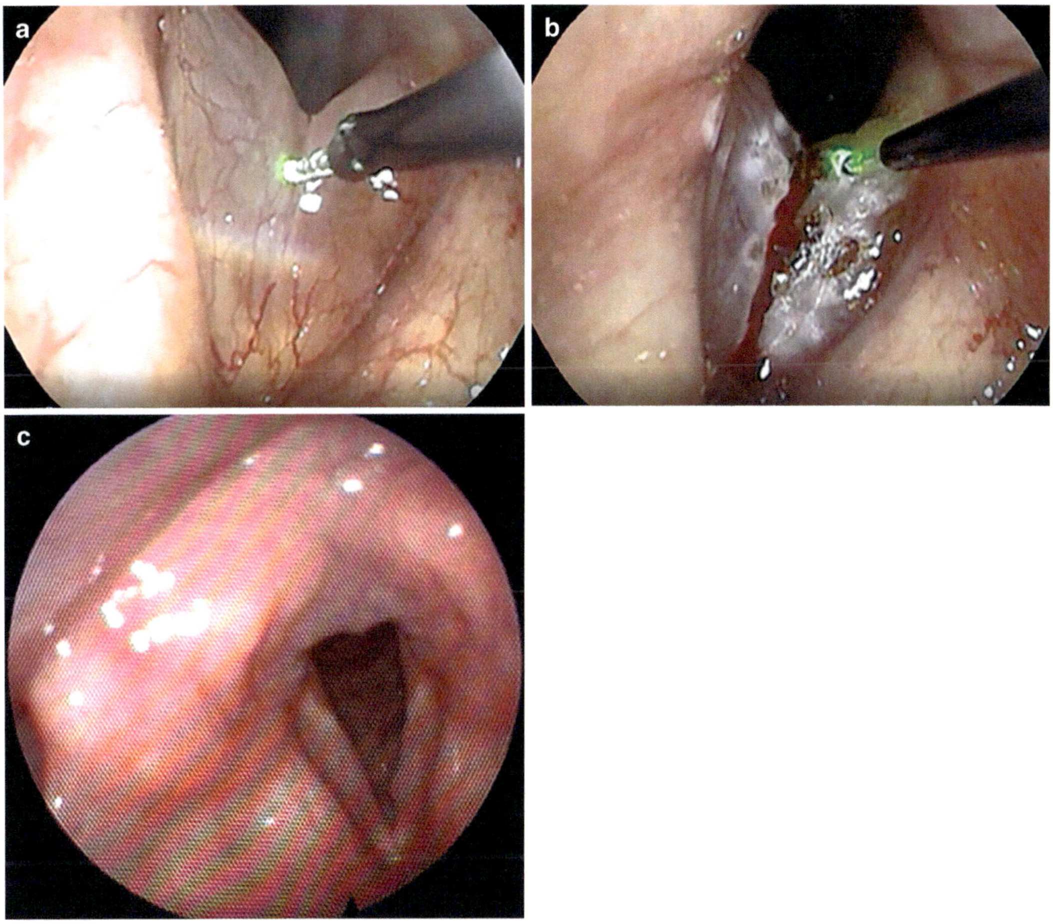

Fig. 4.13 (**a**) An endoscopic view of the larynx showing type 3 Reinke's edema. (**b**) An intraoperative view of the larynx showing the blue laser beam directed toward the left vocal fold. Note blanching of the Reinke's edema bilaterally with partial extrusion of the gelatinous material on the left side. (**c**) A view of the larynx using the flexible nasopharyngoscope 10 weeks after surgery showing complete disease regression on the right side and partial disease regression on the left side

analysis showed an increase in Fo to 177.2 Hz and in HP to 150.4 Hz. On laryngeal examination, she had complete regression of the disease on the left side with mild residual edema of the right vocal fold. Stroboscopic examination showed normal mucosal waves with complete closure of the vocal folds during phonation.

4.2.14 Case 4.14

A 58-year-old female, heavy smoker, presented to the voice clinic (ALH) with deepening of her voice and voice fatigue of few months' duration. The patient denied any history of voice abuse, allergy, or reflux disease. Her Voice Handicap Index-10 (VHI-10) score was 14. Acoustic analysis showed a fundamental frequency (F0) of 119.75 Hz, habitual pitch (HP) of 88.38 Hz, jitter 1.22, shimmer 3.35, a noise-to-harmonics ratio (NHR) of 0.125, and a voice turbulence index (VTI) of 0.049. Aerodynamic parameters revealed a maximum phonation time (MPT) of 6.5 seconds. Laryngeal flexible endoscopic examination revealed bilateral type 3 Reinke's edema (RE) (Fig. 4.14a). The patient underwent

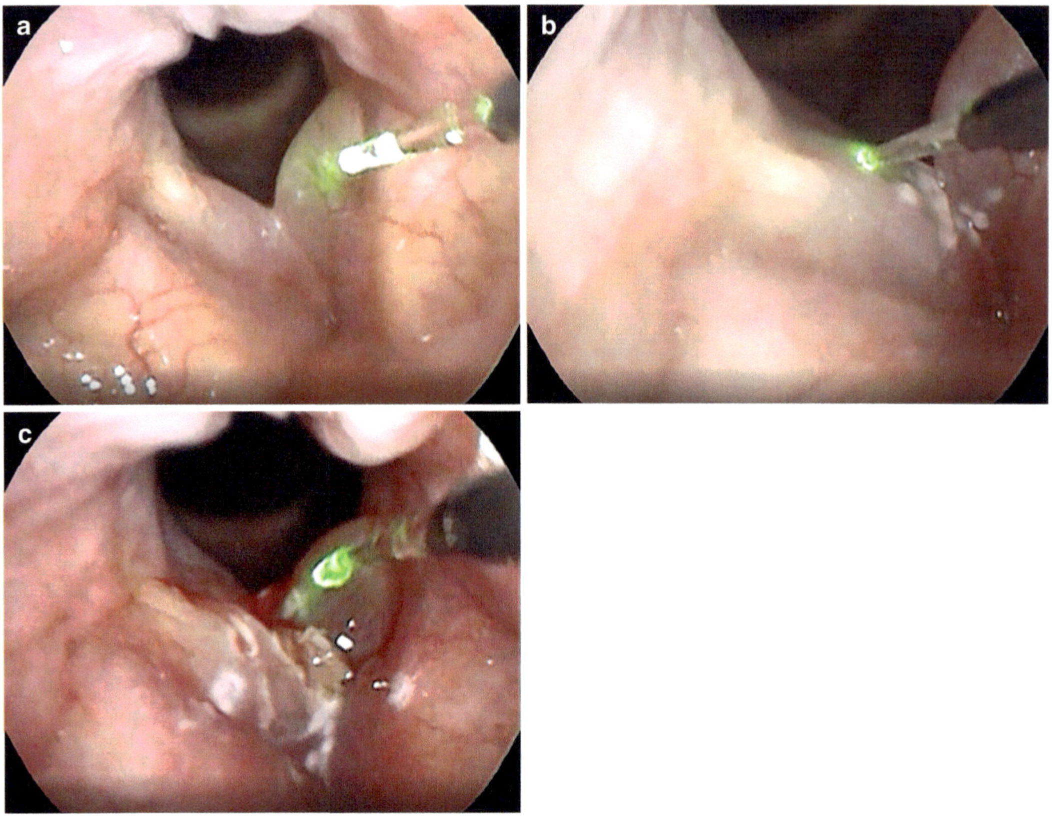

Fig. 4.14 (**a**) An endoscopic view of the larynx showing the bilateral Reinke's edema. Note the contact between the two vocal folds during inspiration. Note also the pachydermia on the interarytenoid mucosal surface. (**b**) An endoscopic view of the larynx showing the blue laser in noncontact mode. Note blanching of the lesion at the site of application of the laser. (**c**) An endoscopic view showing the surgical bed at the end of surgery

office-based blue laser therapy under local anesthesia. The blue laser was introduced into the working channel of the scope, and a total of 115 Joules was delivered (Fig. 4.14b and c). The procedure was tolerated with mild difficulty by the patient, and no significant complications were reported.

4.2.15 Case 4.15

A 41-year-old, female smoker, presented to the Voice Clinic with hoarseness of few years duration. The patient had history of voice abuse and denied any history of allergy or reflux disease. Her Voice Handicap Index-10 (VHI-10) score was 15. Acoustic analysis showed a fundamental frequency (F0) of 185.64 Hz, a habitual pitch (HP) of 196.095 Hz, jitter 1.36, shimmer 1.897, a noise-to-harmonic ratio (NHR) of 0.094, and a voice to turbulence index (VTI) of 0.025. Aerodynamic analysis showed a maximum phonation time (MPT) of 11.86 seconds. Laryngeal examination showed mild Reinke's edema of the right vocal fold (Fig. 4.15).

The patient underwent an office-based blue laser therapy using the contact and noncontact modes (Fig. 4.15b–d). A total of 25.1 Joules was delivered. Following laser therapy, 0.2 ml of dexamethasone (8 mg/2 ml) was injected into the left vocal fold. The procedure was well tolerated by the patient and no complications were noted.

On follow-up 6 weeks later, the patient had marked improvement in her voice quality. Her VHI-10 score dropped to 1. Acoustic analysis showed an increase in F0 to 210.42 Hz, and in HP

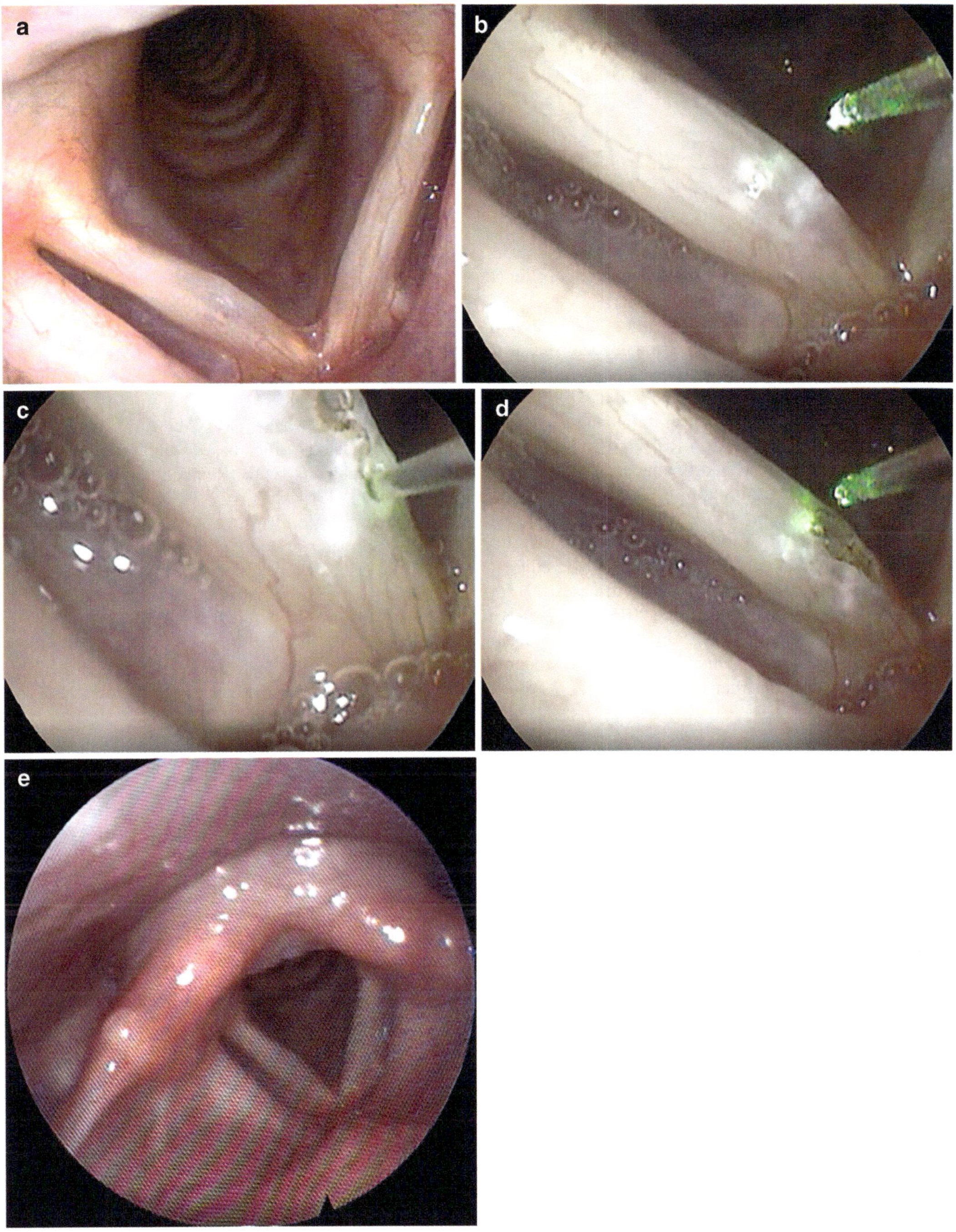

Fig. 4.15 (**a**) An endoscopic view of the larynx showing mild Reinke's edema of the right vocal fold. (**b**) An endoscopic view of the larynx showing the blue laser in non-contact mode. (**c**) An endoscopic view of the larynx showing the blue laser in contact mode. (**d**) An endoscopic view of the larynx showing the surgical bed at the end of blue laser therapy. (**e**) An endoscopic view of the larynx 6 weeks after surgery showing complete regression of the lesion

to 197.97. There was a decrease in jitter to 0.82 and in shimmer to 1.605. Laryngeal examination revealed a complete regression of the lesion (Fig. 4.15e).

References

1. Franco RA, Andrus JG. Common diagnoses and treatments in professional voice users. Otolaryngol Clin N Am. 2007;40(5):1025–61. vii
2. Sataloff RT. Structural abnormalities in the larynx. In: Sataloff RT, editor. Professional voice: the science and art of clinical care. 4th ed. San Diego: Plural Publishing; 2017. p. 1533–67.
3. Koufman JA. Gastroesophageal reflux and voice disorders. In: Rubin JS, Sataloff RS, Korovin GS, Gould WJ, editors. Diagnosis and treatment of voice disorders. New York: Igaku-Shoin; 1995. p. 161–75.
4. Hamdan AL, Sataloff RT, Hawkshaw M. Laryngeal manifestations of gastrointestinal disorders. In: Hamdan AL, Sataloff RT, Hawkshaw MJ, editors. Laryngeal manifestations of systemic diseases. 2018th ed. San Diego: Plural Publishing; 2018. p. 357–541.
5. Hamdan AL, Khalifee E, Abi Akl PR, Ghanem A, El Hage A. Pathogenic role of Reinke's edema in snoring and obstructive sleep apnea. J Voice. 2020;34(3):456–9.
6. Sataloff RT, Chowdhury F, Joglekar S, Hawkshaw MJ. Reinke's edema. In: Sataloff RT, Chowdhury F, Joglekar S, Hawkshaw MJ, editors. Atlas of endoscopic laryngeal surgery. 1st ed. New Delhi: JP Medical Ltd; 2010. p. 91–7.
7. Woo P. Hyaluronidase injection in the vocal folds for vocal hemorrhage, Reinke edema, and hyaluronic acid overinjection: a novel application in the larynx. J Voice. 2018;32(4):492–8.
8. Wang CT, Liao LJ, Cheng PW, Lo WC, Lai MS. Intralesional steroid injection for benign vocal fold disorders: a systematic review and meta-analysis. Laryngoscope. 2013;123(1):197–203.
9. Pitman MJ, Lebowitz-Cooper A, Iacob C, Tan M. Effect of the 532nm pulsed KTP laser in the treatment of Reinke's edema. Laryngoscope. 2012;122(12):2786–92.
10. Hamdan AL, Ghanem A, Abi Akl PR, El Hage A. Unsedated office-based thulium laser therapy in patients with Reinke's edema. J Voice. 2022;36(1):134–9.
11. Lechien JR, Burns JA, Akst LM. The use of 532-nanometer-pulsed potassium-titanyl-phosphate (KTP) laser in laryngology: a systematic review of current indications, safety, and voice outcomes. Ear Nose Throat J. 2021;100(1_suppl):4S–13S.
12. Ghanem A, Hamdan AL. Unsedated office-based blue laser therapy in female patients with Reinke's edema: a retrospective review of 8 cases. J Voice. 2022;36(4):589–97.

5 Office-Based Blue Laser Therapy for Vocal Fold Cysts

5.1 Introduction

Vocal fold cysts are classified as epidermoid cysts or mucus retention cysts (1). On laryngeal examination, the lesion is usually unilateral and well encapsulated, but contralateral reactive lesions are common, and bilateral cysts can occur. Cysts are located on the upper surface of the vocal fold and may protrude onto or originate from its free margin. Epidermoid cysts have a pearl-like appearance whereas mucus retention cysts are yellowish in color (2, 3), or slightly gray. The patient may be asymptomatic or may present with hoarseness and voice fatigue. Treatment often requires surgical removal in addition to voice therapy especially in patients with laryngeal muscle tension and/or vocal fold scars (4–7). Traditionally surgery is performed in the operating room using cold instrumentation, lasers, or both. Complete resection of the lesion is advocated, although marsupialization has been described (8). Office-based laser therapy is a treatment alternative especially for patients at high risk for general anesthesia (9, 10). This chapter presents six cases of vocal fold cysts treated in office using the blue laser.

Supplementary Information The online version contains supplementary material available at https://doi.org/10.1007/978-3-031-71825-0_5.

5.2 Case Presentations

5.2.1 Case 5.1

A 69-year-old female presented to the Voice Clinic (ALH) with a one-year history of hoarseness. The patient denied any history of smoking, voice abuse, or allergy. Her past medical history was positive for gastroesophageal reflux disease that was treated empirically with proton-pump inhibitors. Her Voice Handicap Index-10 (VHI-10) score was 21. Acoustic analysis showed a fundamental frequency (F0) of 144.46 Hz, a habitual pitch (HP) of 159.16 Hz, jitter 1.01, shimmer 2.25, noise-to-harmonic ratio (NHR) of 0.14, and voice turbulence index (VTI) of 0.041. Her maximum phonation time (MPT) was 7.64 seconds. Laryngeal examination revealed a right vocal fold cyst and a reactive lesion on the left vocal fold (Fig. 5.1a). The patient underwent office-based blue laser therapy for the right vocal fold cyst using the 400 micrometer glass fiber. The laser was used initially in noncontact mode to blanch the lesion and then in cutting mode (power 10 W, pulse duration 40 ms, and pulse pause 150 ms) to incise the wall of the cyst (Fig. 5.1b and c). A total of 16.1 Joules was delivered. Following laser therapy, 0.3 ml of dexamethasone (8 mg/2 ml) was injected into the surgical bed, and 0.1 ml was injected into the reactive lesion. The procedure was tolerated well by the patient with no complications noted. On

A. L. Hamdan et al., *Atlas of Office-based Blue Laser Therapy in Laryngology*,
https://doi.org/10.1007/978-3-031-71825-0_5

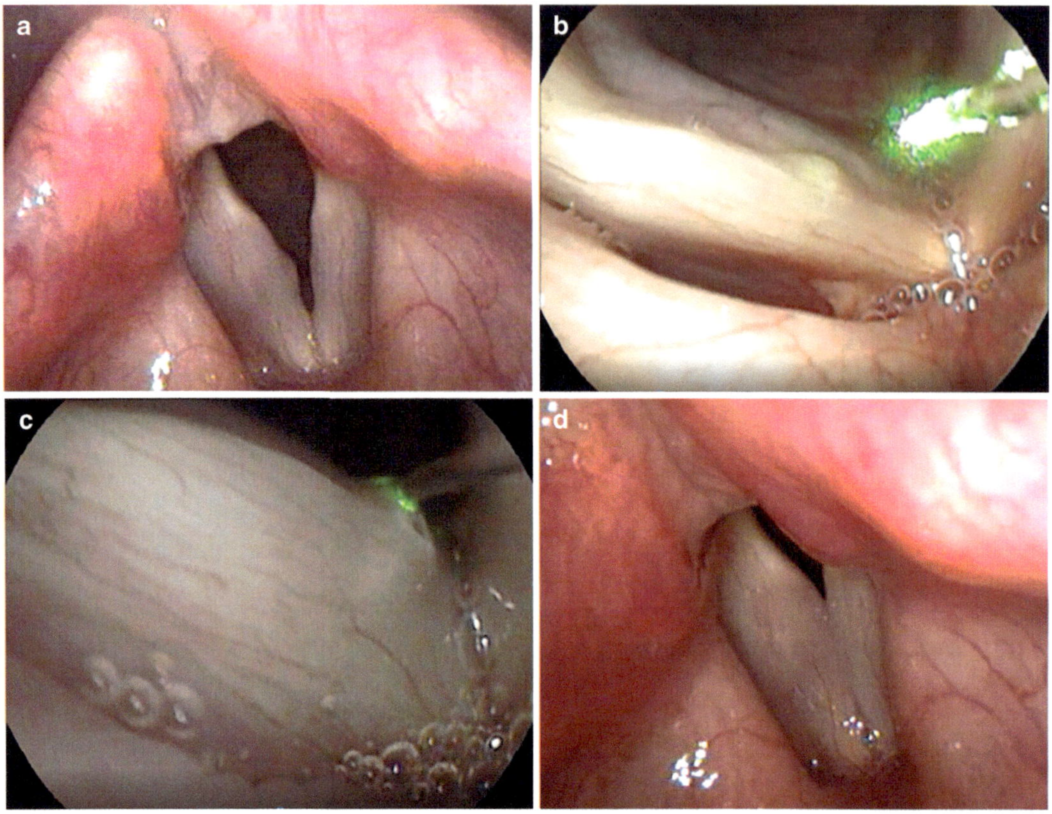

Fig. 5.1 (**a**) An endoscopic view of the larynx showing a right vocal fold cyst. Note the reactive lesion on the opposite vocal fold. (**b**) Intraoperative view of the larynx showing the blue laser beam aiming at the lesion. (**c**) Intraoperative view showing the blue laser glass fiber cutting the wall of the cyst. (**d**) A view of the larynx 4 weeks after surgery showing complete closure of the vocal folds during phonation with regression of the lesion

follow-up 4 weeks later, the patient had substantial improvement in her voice quality. Her VHI-10 score dropped to 2. Acoustic analysis showed an increase in the F0 to 160.73 Hz and in the HP to 164.2 Hz. Laryngeal examination revealed almost complete regression of the lesion with good closure of the vocal folds during phonation (Fig. 5.1d).

5.2.2 Case 5.2

A 60-year-old female, heavy smoker, presented to the Voice Clinic (ALH) with a few months' history of hoarseness. The patient had a history of phonotrauma but denied any allergy or reflux disease. Her Voice Handicap Index-10 (VHI-10) score was 22. Acoustic analysis showed a fundamental frequency (F0) of 113.18 Hz, jitter 0.85, shimmer 3.5, noise-to-harmonic ratio (NHR) of 0.11, and voice turbulence index (VTI) of 0.047. Aerodynamic analysis showed a maximum phonation time (MPT) of 6.2 seconds. Laryngeal endoscopic examination showed a cystic lesion suggestive of an epithelial inclusion cyst on the left vocal fold and a reactive lesion on the right vocal fold (Fig. 5.2a).

The patient underwent office-based blue laser therapy for the left vocal fold cyst using contact and noncontact modes. The laser was used initially in noncontact mode to blanch the lesion, and then the tip of the laser glass fiber was used to create an incision at the upper surface of the lesion in a parallel plane to the vocal fold free edge (Fig. 5.2b and c) (Video 5.1). A total of 12 Joules was delivered. A cup forceps was used to remove the residual disease from the surgical bed (Fig. 5.2d). Following laser therapy, 0.3 ml of

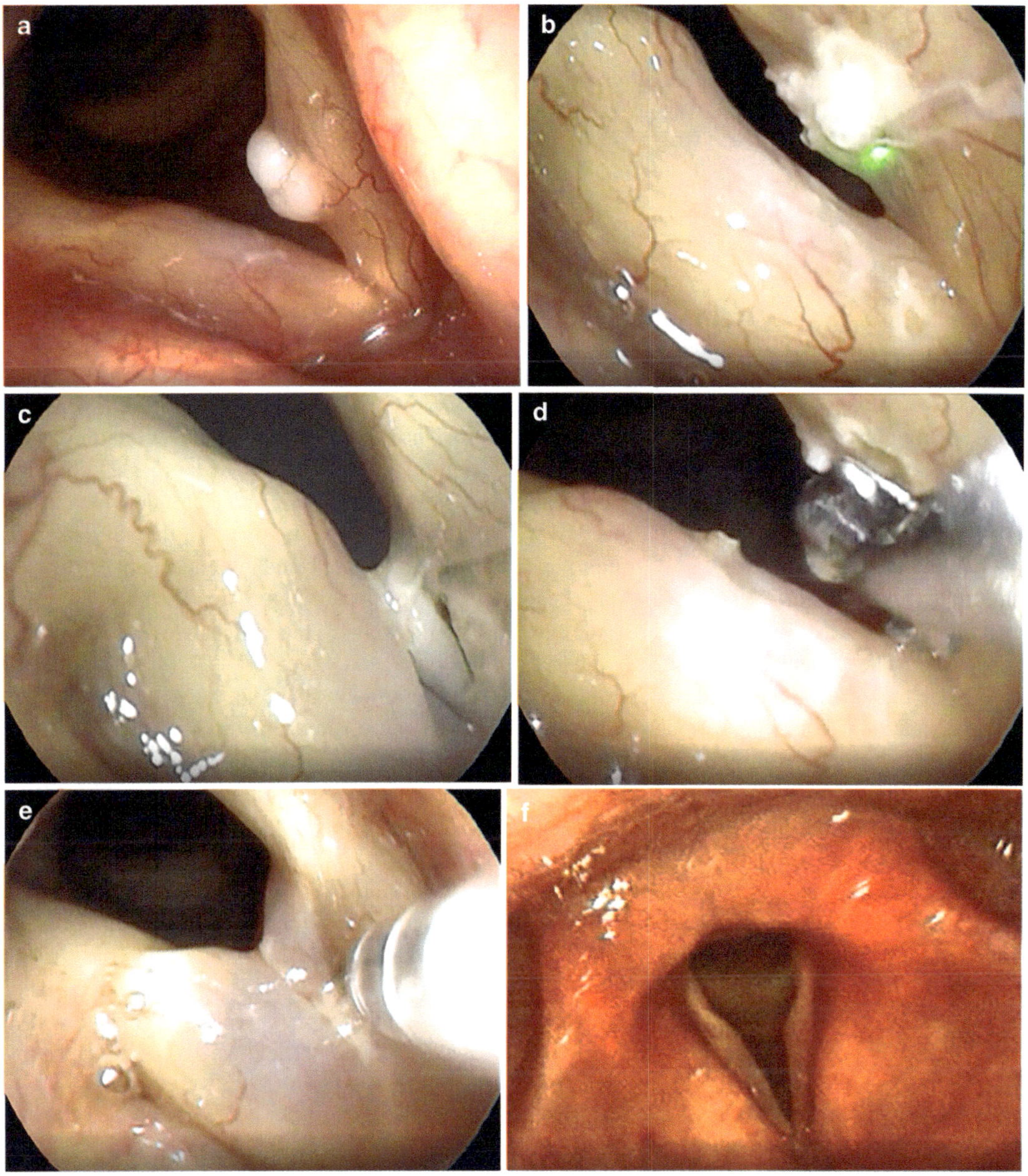

Fig. 5.2 (**a**) An endoscopic view of the larynx showing a left vocal fold subepithelial inclusion cyst. Note the reactive lesion on the right vocal fold. (**b**) Intraoperative view of the larynx showing the laser glass fiber in contact with the lesion. (**c**) An endoscopic view of the larynx showing the incision of the wall of the cyst using the tip of the glass fiber. Note that the plane of incision is parallel to the free edge of the vocal fold. (**d**) The cup forceps was used to remove the content of the cyst and part of its wall. (**e**) An endoscopic view showing injection of 0.2 ml of dexamethasone (8 mg/2 ml) in the left vocal fold using a 25-gauge flexible needle. Note the bleb formation on the left and right vocal fold. (**f**) An endoscopic view of the larynx six weeks after surgery showing complete disease regression

dexamethasone (8 mg/2 ml) was injected into the surgical bed in the left vocal fold, and 0.1 ml was injected into the reactive lesion in the right vocal fold (Fig. 5.2e). The procedure was tolerated well by the patient with no complications noted. On follow-up 6 weeks later, the patient had marked improvement in her voice quality. Her VHI-10 score dropped to 2. Acoustic analysis showed an increase in F0 to 171.16 Hz. Aerodynamic analysis revealed an increase in the MPT to 19.18 seconds. Laryngeal examination revealed complete regression of the lesion (Fig. 5.2f).

5.2.3 Case 5.3

A 59-year-old female, heavy smoker, presented to the Voice Clinic (ALH) with a 2 months history of hoarseness. The patient denied any voice abuse, allergy or reflux disease. Her Voice Handicap Index-10 (VHI-10) score was 14. Acoustic analysis showed a fundamental frequency (F0) of 175.11 Hz, jitter 1.06, shimmer 1.4, a noise-to-harmonic ratio (NHR) of 0.1, and voice turbulence index (VTI) of 0.018. Aerodynamic analysis showed a maximum phonation time (MPT) of 13 seconds. Laryngeal examination revealed a right vocal fold cyst (Fig. 5.3a). The patient underwent office-based blue laser therapy for the right vocal fold cyst using contact and noncontact modes. A total of 25.9 Joules was delivered. Following laser therapy, 0.1 ml of dexamethasone (8 mg/2 ml) was injected into the surgical bed using a 25-gauge flexible needle that was introduced through the working channel of the flexible endoscope (Fig. 5.3b and c; Video 5.2). The procedure was tolerated well by the patient with no complications noted.

On follow-up 3 weeks after surgery, the patient had marked improvement in her voice quality. Her VHI-10 score dropped to 1. Postoperative acoustic analysis showed an increase in the F0 to 181.21 Hz, and laryngeal examination revealed complete regression of the cyst and mild residual edema at the surgical bed (Fig. 5.3d).

5.2.4 Case 5.4

A 31-year-old female, smoker, presented to Voice Clinic (ALH) with a history of hoarseness for a few months. The patient denied any voice abuse, reflux disease or allergy. Her Voice Handicap Index-10 (VHI-10) score was 25. Acoustic analysis showed a fundamental frequency (F0) of 178.2 Hz, habitual pitch (HP) of 187.8 Hz, jitter 1.14, shimmer 2.35, noise-to-harmonic ratio (NHR) of 0.125, and voice turbulence index (VTI) of 0.036. Her maximum phonation time (MPT) was 12.81 seconds. Laryngeal endoscopic examination revealed a right vocal fold pseudocyst with a reactive lesion on the left vocal fold (Fig. 5.4a).

The patient underwent office-based blue laser therapy for her right vocal fold pseudocyst under local anesthesia using power 10 watts, pulse duration 40 ms, and pulse pause 150 ms. A total of 30.3 Joules was delivered during the procedure. The laser was used in contact and noncontact modes (Fig. 5.4b–d; Video 5.3). Following laser therapy, 0.2 ml of dexamethasone (8 mg/2 ml) was injected into the surgical bed, and 0.1 ml was injected into the reactive lesion on the left vocal fold (Fig. 5.4e). The procedure was tolerated well by the patient with no complications noted.

On follow-up 3 weeks later, the patient had marked improvement in her voice quality. Her VHI-10 score dropped to 5. Acoustic analysis postoperatively showed an increase in F0 to 193 Hz and in HP to 195.83 Hz. Her MPT increased to 14.53 seconds. Laryngeal endoscopic examination 3 weeks later showed complete regression of the right vocal fold pseudocyst with persistent mild edema and redness at the site of surgery (Fig. 5.4f). Laryngeal videostroboscopic examination revealed normal mucosal waves. Six weeks later, the laryngeal examination was normal (Fig. 5.4g).

5.2.5 Case 5.5

A 57-year-old male, smoker, presented to the Voice Clinic (ALH) with a change in voice quality of a few months' duration. He had history of voice abuse and overuse. His medical history was positive for gastroesophageal reflux disease that was treated using proton-pump inhibitors. Perceptual voice evaluation revealed severe dysphonia and mild breathiness. His Voice Handicap Index-10 (VHI-10) score was 37. Acoustic and aerodynamic analysis showed a fundamental fre-

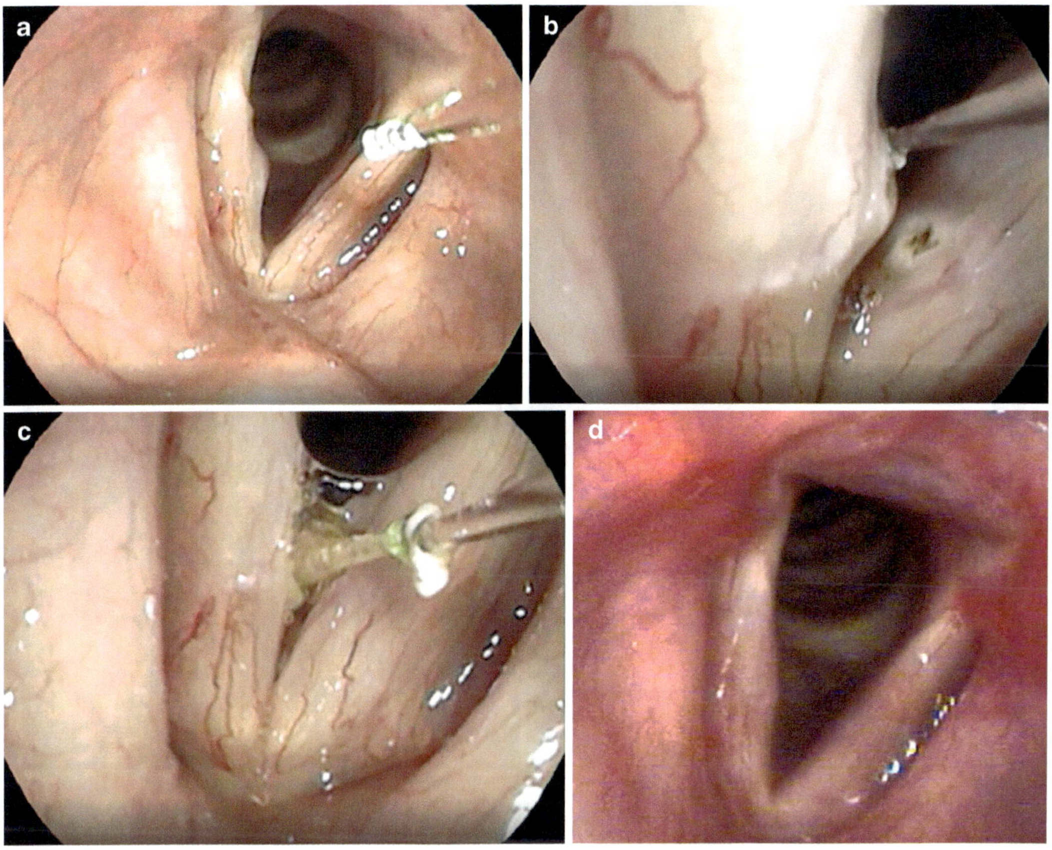

Fig. 5.3 (**a**) An endoscopic view of the larynx showing a right vocal fold cyst. (**b**) Intraoperative view showing the blue laser glass fiber in contact with the wall of the cyst. Note an aberrant strike of the laser on the left vocal fold opposite to the lesion. (**c**) Intraoperative view showing mucopurulent discharge following incision of the wall of the right vocal fold cyst. (**d**) Three weeks after surgery, laryngeal examination showed complete regression of the lesion with only mild residual edema at the surgical bed

quency (F_0) of 159.02 Hz, habitual pitch (HP) of 149.48 Hz, jitter 1.87, shimmer 6.33, noise-to-harmonic ratio (NHR) of 0.148, and voice turbulence index (VTI) of 0.066. His maximum phonation time (MPT) was 8.83 seconds. Laryngeal examination showed a right vocal fold cyst (Fig. 5.5a). On stroboscopic examination, there was a decrease in mucosal wave at the site of the lesion with incomplete closure of the vocal folds during phonation. The patient underwent office-based blue laser therapy using the following settings: power 10 W, pulse duration 40 ms, and pulse pause of 150 ms (Fig. 5.5b; Video 5.4). The laser therapy was followed by steroid injection using 0.1 ml of dexamethasone (8 mg/2 ml). On follow-up 12 weeks later, there was complete regression of the lesion with subjective improvement in voice quality. The patient's VHI-10 score dropped to 0. Acoustic analysis showed a F_0 of 124.0 Hz, HP of 109.9 Hz, jitter 0.83, shimmer 1.83, NHR of 0.12, and VTI of 0.037. His MPT increased to 18.61 seconds. Laryngeal videostroboscopic examination showed complete regression of the lesion with good closure of the vocal folds during phonation (Fig. 5.5c).

5.2.6 Case 5.6

A 45-year-old male, smoker, presented to the Voice Clinic (ALH) with a few years' history of hoarseness. The patient had a history of reflux

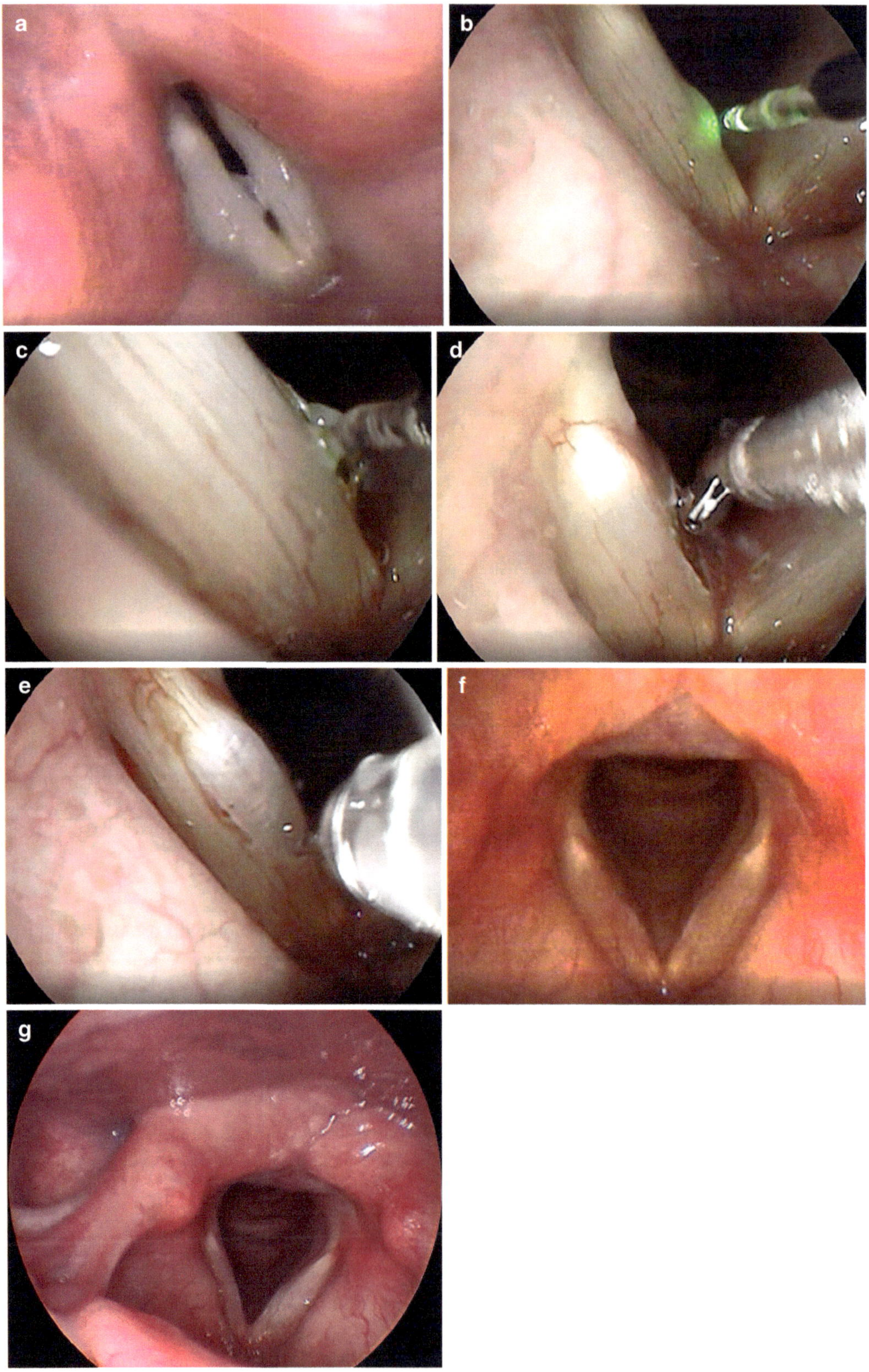
a
b
c
d
e
f
g

Fig. 5.4 (**a**) An endoscopic view of the larynx showing a right vocal fold pseudocyst. Note the incomplete closure of the vocal folds during phonation. (**b**) Intraoperative image of the larynx showing the blue laser glass fiber directed toward the lesion. (**c**) Intra-op view of the larynx showing the blue laser glass fiber incising the wall of the pseudocyst. Note the yellowish discharge coming out from the cyst. (**d**) Intraoperative view of the larynx showing removal of the surgical debris using a cup forceps after the blue laser therapy. (**e**) An endoscopic view showing the injection of 0.2 ml of dexamethasone (8 mg/2 ml). Note the bleb at the site of injection confirming that the injection was made in the superficial layer of the lamina propria. (**f**) Postoperative view of the vocal folds 3 weeks after office-based blue laser surgery showing complete regression of the lesion with residual edema and redness at the site of surgery. (**g**) Laryngeal examination 6 weeks after surgery showing complete regression of the lesion

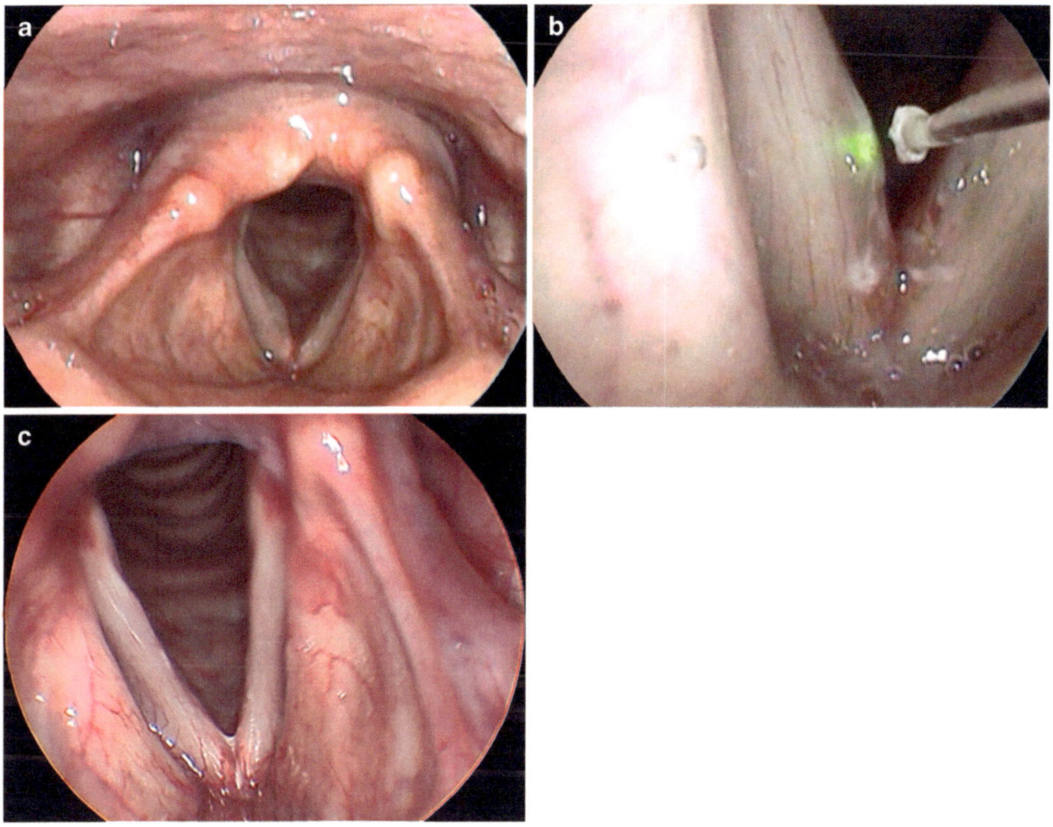

Fig. 5.5 (**a**) An endoscopic view of the larynx showing a right vocal fold cystic lesion occupying almost half of the vocal fold. (**b**) An endoscopic view showing the blue laser glass fiber aiming at the lesion. Note the aberrant strikes anteriorly. (**c**) Follow-up examination 3 months after surgery showing complete regression of the lesion

disease but no history of allergy. His Voice Handicap Index-10 (VHI-10) score was 3. Acoustic analysis showed a fundamental frequency (F0) of 105.28 Hz, habitual pitch (HP) of 93 Hz, jitter 0.473, shimmer 1.824, noise-to-harmonic ration (NHR) of 0.144, and voice turbulence index (VTI) of 0.048. His maximum phonation time (MPT) was 20.14 seconds. Laryngeal examination revealed a cyst on the right vocal fold and a reactive lesion on the left vocal fold (Fig. 5.6a). The patient underwent office-based blue laser therapy for the right vocal fold cyst using contact and noncontact modes. A total of 34.6 Joules was delivered (Fig. 5.6b and c; Video 5.5). Following laser therapy, 0.1 ml of dexamethasone (8 mg/2 ml) was injected into the right vocal fold, and 0.1 ml was injected into the reactive lesion on the contralateral side. The pro-

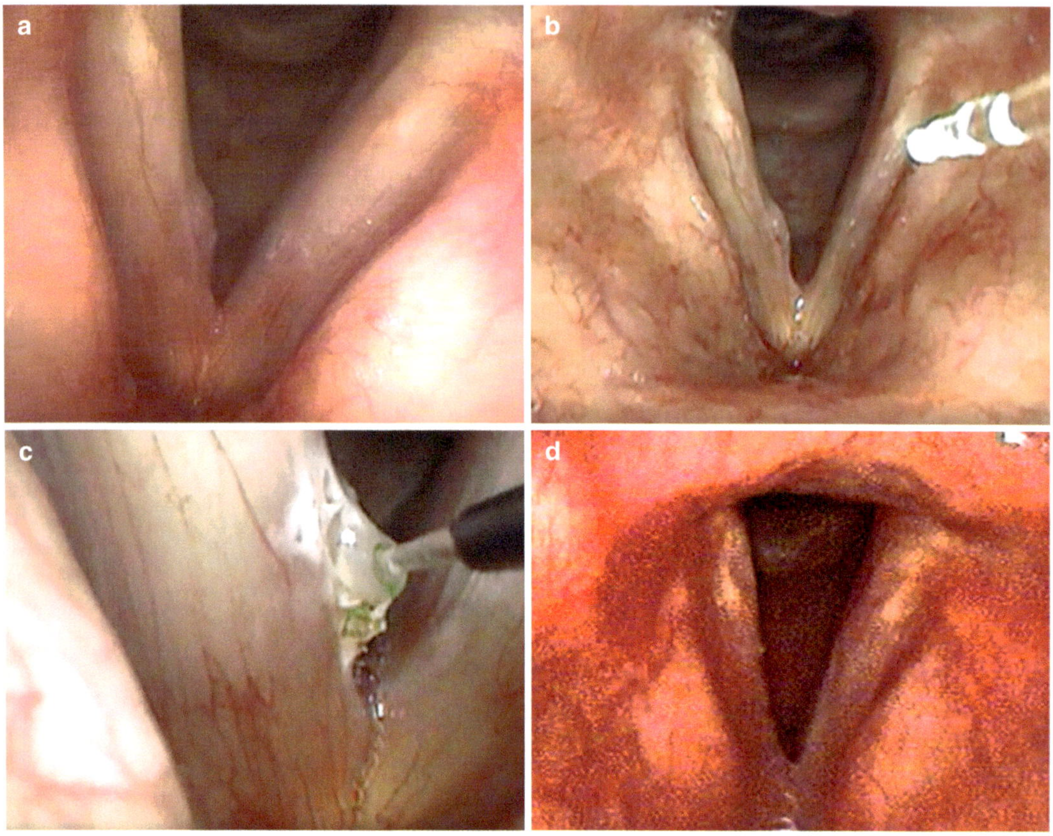

Fig. 5.6 (**a**) An endoscopic view of the larynx showing a cyst on the free margin of the right vocal fold and a reactive lesion on the left vocal fold. (**b**) An endoscopic view of the larynx showing the blue laser glass fiber directed toward the right vocal fold cyst. (**c**) An intraoperative view of the larynx showing the tip of the blue laser glass fiber inserted into the lumen of the cyst. Note the mucus content extruding from the cyst. (**d**) A postoperative view of the larynx three weeks after surgery showing almost complete regression of the lesion. Note the irregular free margin of the right vocal fold

cedure was tolerated well by the patient with no complications noted. The patient presented 3 weeks after surgery with marked improvement in his voice quality. On examination he had almost complete regression of the lesion (Fig. 5.6d).

References

1. Rosen CA, Gartner-Schmidt J, Hathaway B, Simpson CB, Postma GN, Courey M, et al. A nomenclature paradigm for benign midmembranous vocal fold lesions. Laryngoscope. 2012;122(6):1335–41.
2. Naunheim MR, Carroll TL. Benign vocal fold lesions: update on nomenclature, cause, diagnosis, and treatment. Curr Opin Otolaryngol Head Neck Surg. 2017;25(6):453–8.
3. Franco RA, Andrus JG. Common diagnoses and treatments in professional voice users. Otolaryngol Clin N Am. 2007;40(5):1025–61. vii
4. Courey MS, Gardner GM, Stone RE, Ossoff RH. Endoscopic vocal fold microflap: a three-year experience. Ann Otol Rhinol Laryngol. 1995;104(4 Pt 1):267–73.
5. Bouchayer M, Cornut G. Microsurgical treatment of benign vocal fold lesions: indications, technique, results. Folia Phoniatr (Basel). 1992;44(3–4):155–84.
6. Sataloff RT, Farhad C, Shruti J. Vocal fold cysts. In: Sataloff RT, Chowdhury F, Joglekar S, Hawkshaw

MJ, editors. Atlas of endoscopic laryngeal surgery. 1st ed. New Delhi: JP Medical Ltd; 2011. p. 59–68.

7. Hsu CM, Armas GL, Su CY. Marsupialization of vocal fold retention cysts: voice assessment and surgical outcomes. Ann Otol Rhinol Laryngol. 2009;118(4):270–5.
8. Hamdan AL, Rizk SA. Unsedated office-based thulium laser therapy in patients with vocal fold cysts. Ear Nose Throat J. 2021;100(1):NP39.
9. Gao WZ, Abu-Ghanem S, Reder LS, Amin M, Johns MM. A novel approach to vocal fold mucous retention cysts: awake KTP laser-assisted marsupialization. J Voice. 2022;36(4):570–3.
10. Hamdan AL, Abou Raji Feghali P, Hosri J, Ghanem A, Alam E. Office-based laser therapy for vocal fold cyst: a promising alternative therapy using the 445 nm blue laser. J Voice. 2023;19:S0892-1997(23)00172-8.

6 Office-Based Blue Laser Therapy of Vocal Fold Varices and Other Vascular Lesions

6.1 Introduction

Vocal fold varices and ectasias are aberrant microvasculature lesions of the vocal folds. The etiology is complex. Phonotrauma with an increase in capillary pressure is thought to be the main precipitating factor [1]. Other risk factors include laryngopharyngeal reflux disease and fluctuation in sex hormones [2]. Vocal fold varices and ectasias are located commonly on the upper surface or striking zone of the vocal fold [3]. Affected patients may be asymptomatic or may complain of hoarseness. The change in voice quality can be secondary to the mass effect of the lesion (which can fluctuate with vascular engorgement) or to increased stiffness in the vocal fold secondary to hemorrhage. The main indication for surgery is persistent dysphonia with impairment in mucosal waves seen on laryngeal videostroboscopy. Another relative indication is recurrent vocal fold hemorrhage [4]. Surgical removal of the lesion or thermolysis is usually performed in the operating room under general anesthesia. With the advances in technology, different types of photoangiolytic lasers have been used in-office to achieve disease regression [5–7]. This chapter describes office-based blue laser therapy for vocal fold varices and ectasias.

Supplementary Information The online version contains supplementary material available at https://doi.org/10.1007/978-3-031-71825-0_6.

6.2 Case Presentations

6.2.1 Case 6.1

A 37-year-old male, smoker, presented to the Voice Clinic (ALH) with hoarseness of a few months' duration. The patient had history of voice abuse and denied any history of allergy or reflux disease. His Voice Handicap Index-10 (VHI-10) score was 7. Acoustic analysis showed a fundamental frequency (F0) of 151.36 Hz, habitual pitch (HP) of 127.09 Hz, jitter 0.65, shimmer 2.08, a noise-to-harmonic ratio (NHR) of 0.14, and a voice turbulence index (VTI) of 0.033. His maximum phonation time (MPT) was 14.4 seconds. Laryngeal flexible endoscopic examination revealed a vascular lesion on the upper surface of the left vocal fold and white mucosa suggestive of a mucosal tear. Voice rest was advised and prednisolone 40 mg/day was prescribed. Laryngeal examination three weeks later showed no significant improvement (Fig. 6.1a). The patient underwent office-based blue laser therapy using the noncontact mode (Fig. 6.1b; Video 6.1). Laser setting was power 2 watts, pulse duration 10 ms, and pulse pause 300 ms. This was followed by injection of 0.1–0.2 ml of dexamethasone (8 mg/2 ml) at the site of the lesion. The procedure was tolerated well by the patient with no complications noted. On follow up 2 months later, the patient had marked improvement in his voice quality. His VHI-10 score was 4. There was no significant

A. L. Hamdan et al., *Atlas of Office-based Blue Laser Therapy in Laryngology*,
https://doi.org/10.1007/978-3-031-71825-0_6

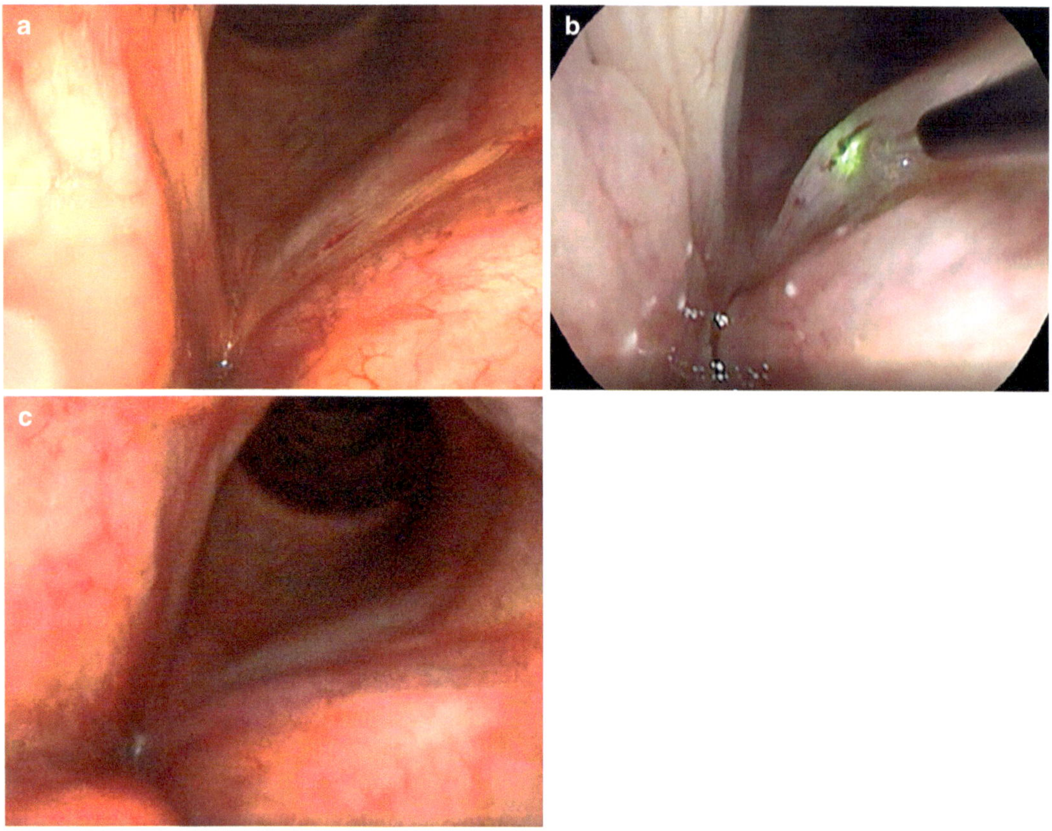

Fig. 6.1 (**a**) A pre-operative view of the larynx showing dilated microvasculature on the upper surface of the right vocal fold with adjacent white mucosa suggestive of a mucosal tear. (**b**) Intraoperative view of the larynx showing the blue laser glass fiber in noncontact mode directed toward the dilated microvasculature of the left vocal fold. (**c**) An endoscopic view of the larynx 2 months after surgery showing complete regression of the dilated vessel on the upper surface of the left vocal fold and resolution of the white discoloration of the mucosa

change in jitter and shimmer (0.61 and 2.45, respectively). Laryngeal examination showed complete regression of the dilated vessel (Fig. 6.1c).

6.2.2 Case 6.2

A 48-year-old female presented to the Voice Clinic (ALH) with hoarseness of a few months' duration. The patient had a history of voice abuse and denied any history of smoking, allergy, or reflux disease. Laryngeal endoscopic examination revealed a hemorrhagic lesion on the upper surface of the right vocal fold, with a reactive lesion on the left vocal fold (Fig. 6.2a). The patient underwent office-based blue laser therapy under local anesthesia using contact and noncontact modes (Fig. 6.2b–e; Video 6.2). A total of 57.2 Joules was delivered. The cup forceps was used to remove the remaining lesion after ablation. Following laser therapy, 0.1 ml of dexamethasone (8 mg/2 ml) was injected at the surgical site. The procedure was tolerated well by the patient with no complications noted.

6.2.3 Case 6.3

A 35-year-old female, smoker, presented to the Voice Clinic (ALH) with a history of intermittent hoarseness. The patient had a history of phonotrauma and denied any history of allergy or reflux disease. Her Voice Handicap Index-10 (VHI-10)

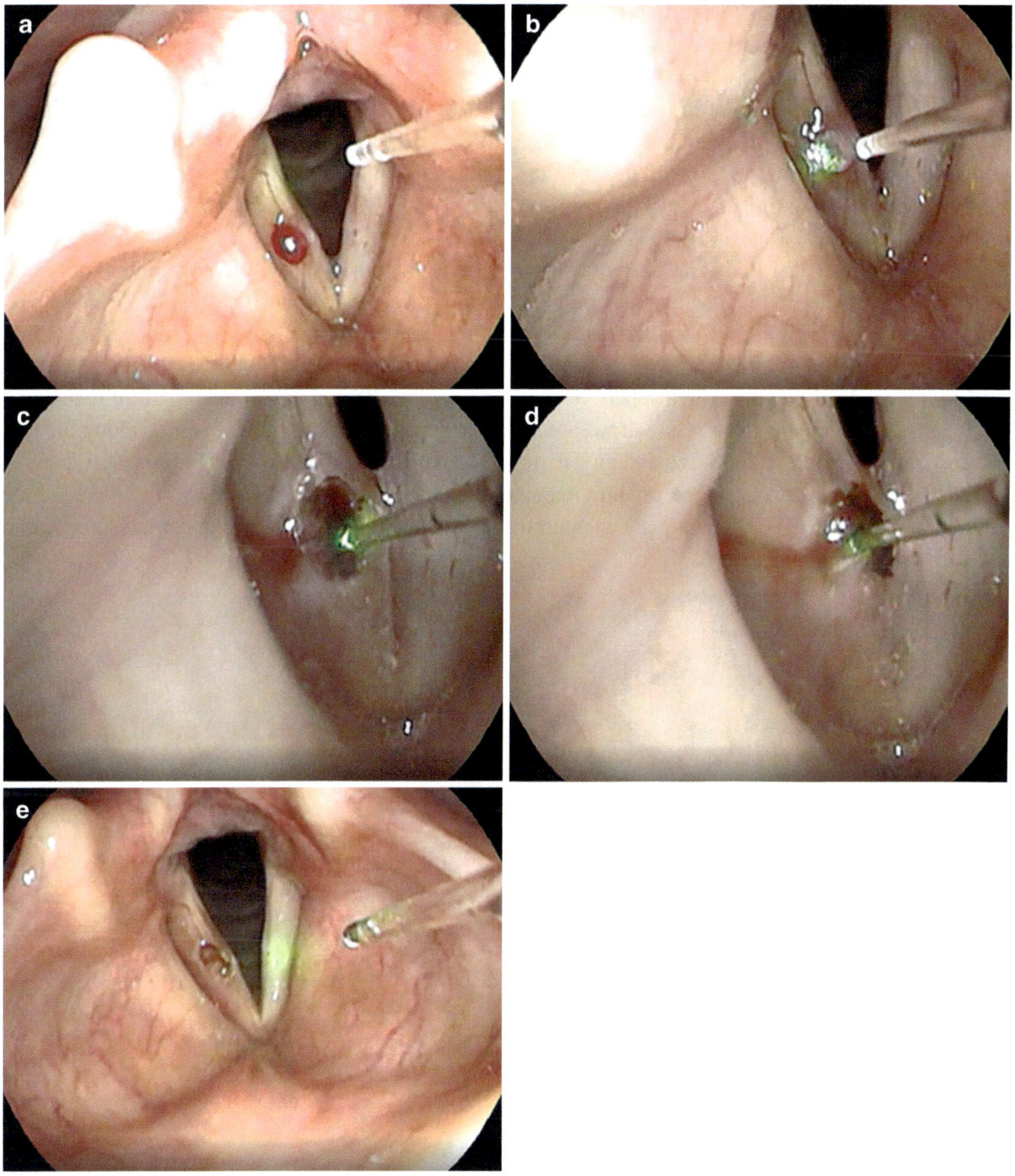

Fig. 6.2 (**a**) An endoscopic view of the larynx showing the hemorrhagic lesion on the upper surface of the right vocal fold. Note the reactive lesion on the free edge of the left vocal fold. (**b**) An endoscopic view of the larynx showing the blue laser glass fiber in noncontact mode. Note blanching of the lesion at the site of the laser beam. (**c**) An image showing the blue laser glass fiber in contact mode against the lesion. (**d**) An endoscopic view of the larynx showing how the blue laser glass fiber is used to peel the lesion following its coagulation. (**e**) An image showing complete regression of the lesion with discoloration at the end of surgery

score was 24. Acoustic analysis showed a fundamental frequency (F0) of 181.03 Hz, habitual pitch (HP) of 181.88 Hz, jitter 1.1, shimmer 1.97, a noise-to-harmonic ratio (NHR) of 0.106, and a voice turbulence index (VTI) of 0.033. Her maximum phonation time (MPT) was 6.81 seconds. Laryngeal examination revealed a small hematoma with a hemorrhagic lesion on the left vocal fold (Fig. 6.3a). The patient was advised to observe voice rest, and was given a 10-day course of prednisolone, following which she had only mild improvement in her voice quality. The patient underwent office-based blue laser therapy for the left vocal fold vascular lesion, and a total of 12.4 Joules was delivered (Fig. 6.3b). Following laser therapy, 0.2 ml of dexamethasone (8 mg/2 ml) was injected into the surgical bed of the left vocal fold and into the reactive lesion of the right vocal fold. The procedure was tolerated well by the patient with no complications noted. On follow-up 6 weeks later, the patient had marked improvement in her voice quality. Her VHI-10 score dropped to 5. Postoperative acoustic analysis showed an increase in the F0 to 185.58 Hz and in HP to 185.24 Hz. There was a decrease in shimmer to 1.67, and in the VTI to 0.025. Her MPT increased to 8 seconds. Laryngeal examination revealed residual swelling of the surgical bed. The patient was advised to undergo voice therapy (Fig. 6.3c).

6.2.4 Case 6.4

A 41-year-old male presented to the Voice Clinic (ALH) with hoarseness of few months' duration. The patient had a history of voice abuse and denied any history of smoking, allergy, or reflux disease. His Voice Handicap Index (VHI-10) score was 20. Laryngeal examination revealed a hemorrhagic lesion (dilated vessel) along the free edge of the right vocal fold (Fig. 6.4a).

The patient underwent office-based blue laser therapy using the near-contact mode, and

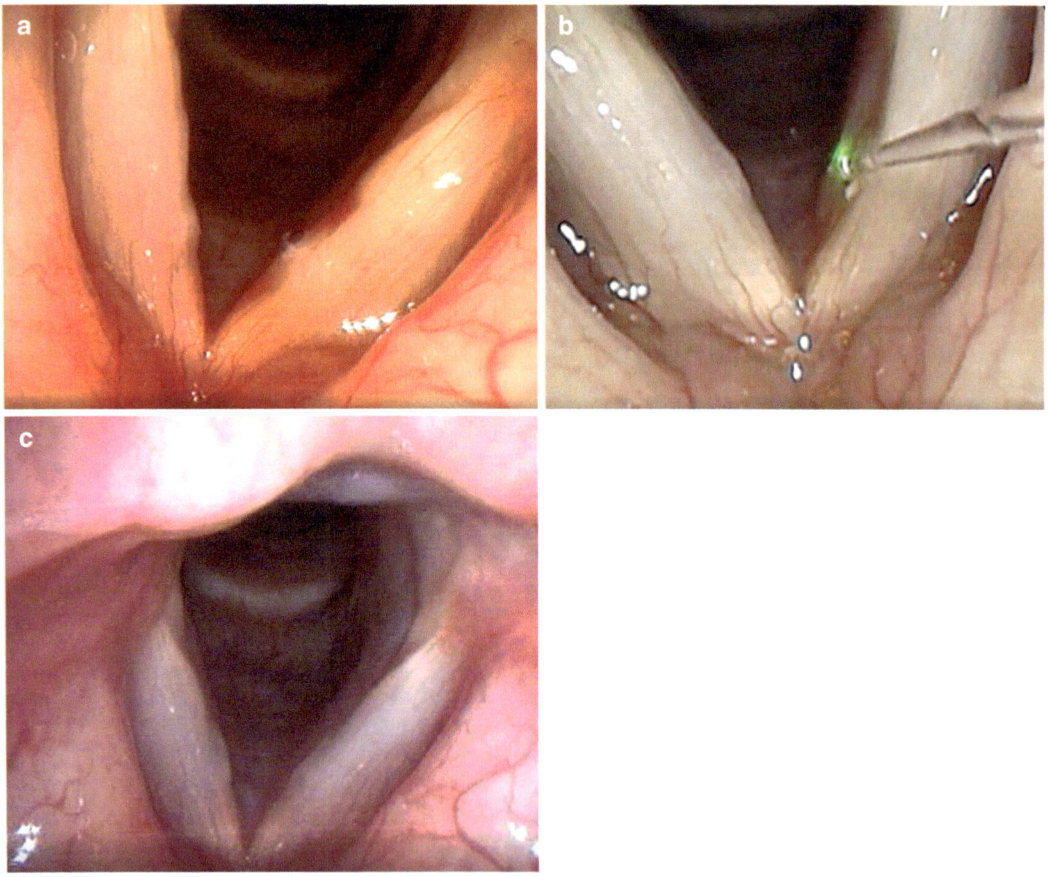

Fig. 6.3 (**a**) Laryngeal endoscopy showing a small hematoma and a hemorrhagic lesion on the left vocal fold. Note the reactive lesion on the right vocal fold. Note a reactive lesion on the right vocal fold. (**b**) Intraoperative view of the larynx showing the blue laser glass fiber (400 micrometer) targeting the lesion in near-contact mode. (**c**) A postoperative view of the larynx 6 weeks after surgery showing complete regression of the lesion

a total of 13.7 Joules was delivered (Fig. 6.4b and c; Video 6.3). The procedure was tolerated well by the patient with no complications noted. On follow-up 6 weeks later, the patient had marked improvement in his voice quality. His VHI-10 score dropped to 4. Laryngeal examination revealed complete regression of the lesion.

6.2.5 Case 6.5

A 68-year-old male, smoker, presented to the Voice Clinic (ALH) with hoarseness of a few months' duration. The patient had history of voice abuse and denied any history of smoking, reflux disease, or allergy. His Voice Handicap Index (VHI-10) score was 22. Acoustic analysis showed a fundamental frequency (F0) of 172.51 Hz, habitual pitch (HP) of 173.71 Hz, jitter 1.8, shimmer 3.27, a noise-to-harmonic ratio (NHR) of 0.091, and a voice turbulence index (VTI) of 0.044. Aerodynamic analysis showed a maximum phonation time (MPT) of 17.73 seconds. Laryngeal flexible endoscopic examination revealed a right vocal fold hemorrhagic lesion and a reactive lesion on the left vocal fold (Fig. 6.5a).

The patient underwent office-based blue laser therapy using the 400 micrometers glass fiber in noncontact mode (Fig. 6.5b; Video 6.4). The lesion disappeared toward the end of surgery (Fig. 6.5c). The procedure was tolerated well by the patient with no complications noted. On follow-up 4 weeks later, the patient had improvement in his voice quality. His VHI-10 score

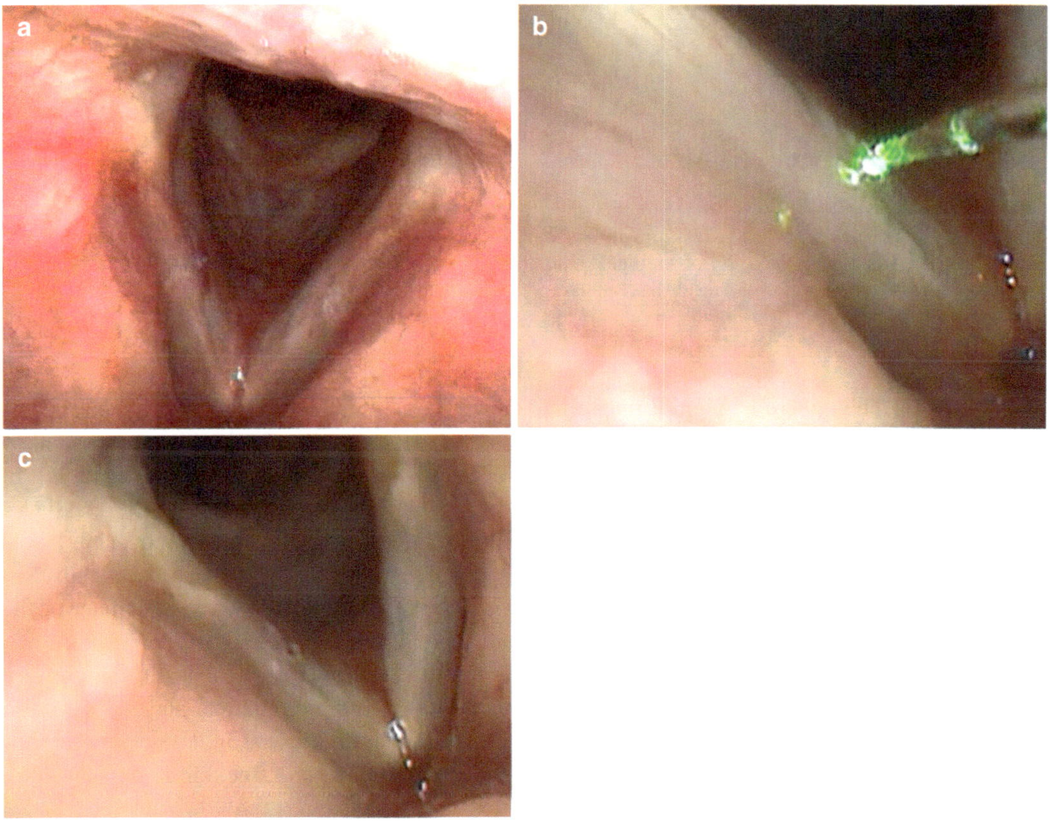

Fig. 6.4 (**a**) An endoscopic view of the larynx showing a right vocal fold dilated vessel. Note the punctate mass near the middle. (**b**) An endoscopic view of the larynx showing the blue laser glass fiber in near-contact mode. (**c**) An endoscopic view of the larynx toward the end of surgery showing blanching and complete regression of the lesion

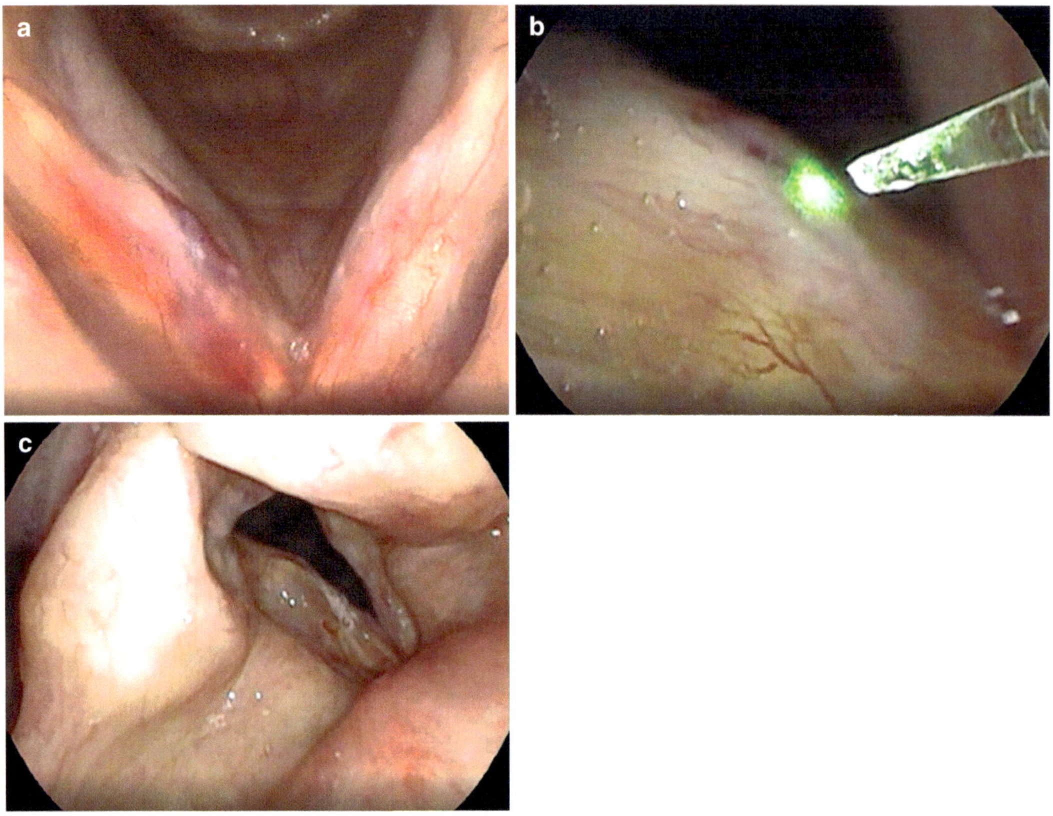

Fig. 6.5 (**a**) An endoscopic view of the larynx showing a right vocal fold hemorrhagic lesion fusiform in shape, involving almost the entire lower lip of the vocal fold. Note the yellowish discoloration and residual submucosal hematoma. (**b**) An endoscopic view of the larynx showing the blue laser glass fiber in noncontact mode. Note blanching of the lesion. (**c**) An endoscopic view toward the end of surgery showing complete regression and blanching of the lesion

dropped to 13. There were no significant differences in the acoustic and aerodynamic analyses. Laryngeal examination on follow-up (4 weeks later) revealed complete regression of the lesion except for mild edema and inflammation at the site of the surgery.

6.2.6 Case 6.6

This 36-year-old male singer presented with a history of laryngopharyngeal reflux (LPR) and dysphonia despite having had multiple voice therapy sessions. His dysphonia was related primarily to the right vocal fold mass (which looked vascular) and glottic insufficiency (Fig. 6.6a). In the operating room, exposure of the mass was limited even with an anterior commissure laryngoscope, and the mass could be reduced only partially with a blue laser. Two months later in the office, blue laser was used to vaporize the remaining right vocal fold mass. The settings used were 6 watts, 40 ms pulse duration, and 300 ms pulse pause (Fig. 6.6b; Video 6.5). The mass was substantially reduced one week after the procedure (Fig. 6.6c).

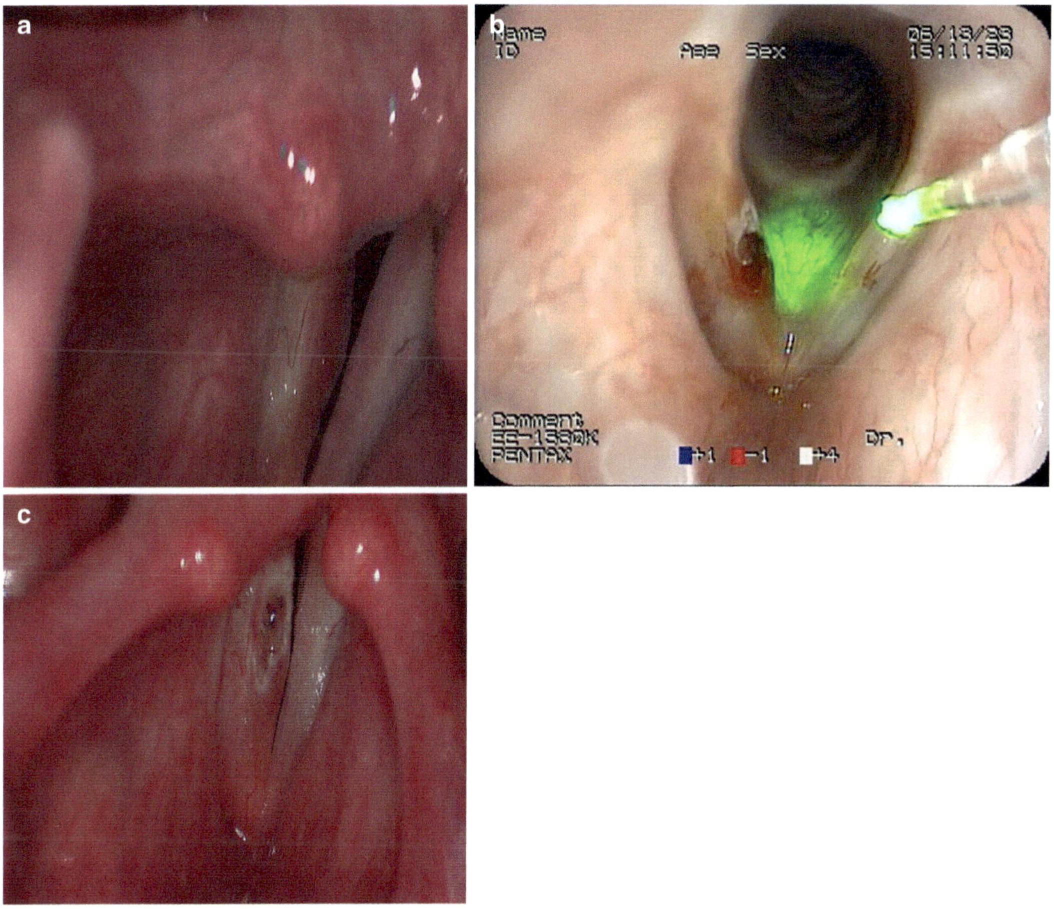

Fig. 6.6 (**a**) Laryngeal examination showing right vocal fold mass. (**b**) In office blue laser was used primarily in non-contact mode to vaporize the right vocal fold mass. (**c**) Laryngeal examination one week after procedure

References

1. Austin S, Divi V, Hawkshaw M, Sataloff RT. Vocal fold varicosities. Ear Nose Throat J. 2011;90(2):56–7.
2. Newman SR, Butler J, Hammond EH, Gray SD. Preliminary report on hormone receptors in the human vocal fold. J Voice. 2000;14(1):72–81.
3. Hochman I, Sataloff RT, Hillman RE, Zeitels SM. Ectasias and varices of the vocal fold: clearing the striking zone. Ann Otol Rhinol Laryngol. 1999;108(1):10–6.
4. Sataloff RT. Patient history. In: Sataloff RT, editor. Professional voice: the science and art of clinical care. 4th ed. San Diego: Plural Publishing; 2017. p. 363–86.
5. Hsiung MW, Kang BH, Su WF, Pai L, Wang HW. Clearing microvascular lesions of the true vocal fold with the KTP/532 laser. Ann Otol Rhinol Laryngol. 2003;112(6):534–9.
6. Zeitels SM, Akst LM, Burns JA, Hillman RE, Broadhurst MS, Anderson RR. Pulsed angiolytic laser treatment of ectasias and varices in singers. Ann Otol Rhinol Laryngol. 2006;115(8):571–80.
7. Miller BJ, Abdelhamid A, Karagama Y. Applications of office-based 445 nm blue laser transnasal flexible laser surgery: a case series and review of practice. Ear Nose Throat J. 2021;100(1_suppl):105S–12S.

7 Office-Based Blue Laser Therapy for Vocal Fold Granuloma

7.1 Introduction

Vocal fold granuloma is a benign lesion that grows following injury to the mucosal lining of the vocal fold or process [1]. An inflammatory cascade is triggered leading to ulceration and mass formation. The most common causes are trauma and laryngopharyngeal reflux disease. The trauma can be secondary to intubation, may occur following phonosurgery [2, 3], or may be phonotrauma. Patients with vocal process granuloma may be asymptomatic or can present with repetitive throat clearing, globus sensation, dysphagia and a change in voice quality, and occasionally with pain. Hoarseness is the most common presenting symptom [3]. On laryngeal examination, the lesion can be ulcerative, fungating, pedunculated, or sessile. The size of the lesion may vary with the extent of the disease and its duration. Conservative therapy using antireflux medications and behavioral modification may be successful in 50% of the cases. In those who fail conservative therapy, other forms of intervention are needed. Surgery is associated with high recurrence rates [4–6]. Other treatment modalities include laryngeal botulinum toxin injection, steroid injection, and laser therapy [7–11], in addition to voice therapy and intensive reflux management. This chapter describes the use of blue laser for the treatment of vocal fold granuloma in an office setting.

7.2 Case Presentations

7.2.1 Case 7.1

A 46-year-old male presented to the Voice Clinic (ALH) with a history of throat clearing, globus sensation and hoarseness of few months' duration. He had a history of reflux disease that was treated with proton-pump inhibitors intermittently. The patient denied any history of laryngeal surgery or trauma. His Voice Handicap Index-10 (VHI-10) score was 5. On laryngeal examination, he had a left vocal process granuloma. The patient was started on antireflux treatment, steroid inhaler and was advised to undergo voice therapy for three months. On follow up, he had no improvement in his symptoms. Laryngeal examination showed persistence of the left vocal process granuloma. The patient was offered various treatment options, and he elected to undergo office-based biopsy and laser therapy. The surgery was performed in-office using the blue laser in noncontact and contact modes (power 10 watts, pulse duration 40 ms, and pause time 300 ms) (Fig. 7.1a–c; Video 7.1). Following laser surgery, the base of the lesion was injected with 0.2 ml of dexamethasone (8 mg/2 ml). On follow up 12 weeks later, the patient had marked improvement in his voice quality with decrease

Supplementary Information The online version contains supplementary material available at https://doi.org/10.1007/978-3-031-71825-0_7.

A. L. Hamdan et al., *Atlas of Office-based Blue Laser Therapy in Laryngology*,
https://doi.org/10.1007/978-3-031-71825-0_7

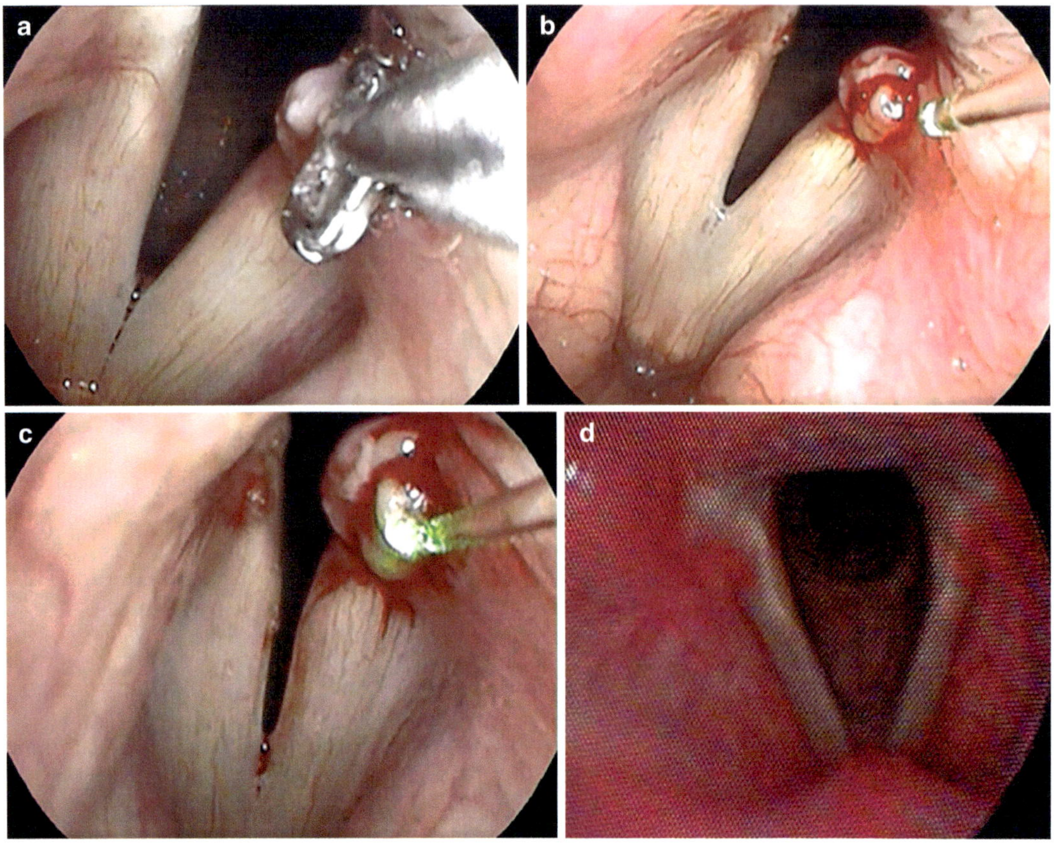

Fig. 7.1 (**a**) A laryngeal view of the larynx showing biopsy of the left vocal process granuloma. (**b**) An endoscopic view of the larynx showing the blue laser glass fiber aiming at the left vocal fold granuloma. (**c**) An endoscopic view of the larynx showing the blue laser glass fiber in contact with the left vocal process granuloma. (**d**) An endoscopic view 3 months post-surgery showing complete regression of the lesion

in his VHI-10 score to 0. On laryngeal examination, he had complete resolution of the lesion (Fig. 7.1d). The patient was advised to stay on antireflux treatment for 3 more months, after which he was to be reevaluated.

7.2.2 Case 7.2

A 30-year-old male with a history of papillary thyroid carcinoma presented to the Voice Clinic (ALH) with hoarseness and repetitive throat clearing of 2 months' duration. His symptoms had started 2 weeks following total thyroidectomy and neck dissection. His VHI-10 score was 36. On laryngeal examination, he had a right vocal process granuloma (Fig. 7.2a). The patient underwent office-based blue laser therapy using contact and noncontact modes. The laser setting was power 10 W, pulse duration 40 ms, and pulse pause 300 ms (Video 7.2). The laser procedure was followed by steroid injection, 0.1–2 ml of dexamethasone 8 mg/2 ml (Figure 7.2b–d). On follow up 3 months later, he had marked improvement in his symptoms. His VHI-10 score decreased to 14. On laryngeal examination he had complete resolution of his lesion (Fig. 7.2e). The patient was reassured and kept on antireflux treatment for 3 months, after which he was to be reevaluated.

7.2.3 Case 7.3

An 18-year-old woman with history of laryngopharyngeal reflux (LPR) presented to us (RTS) with dysphonia despite having had multiple voice therapy sessions. The patient had completed a

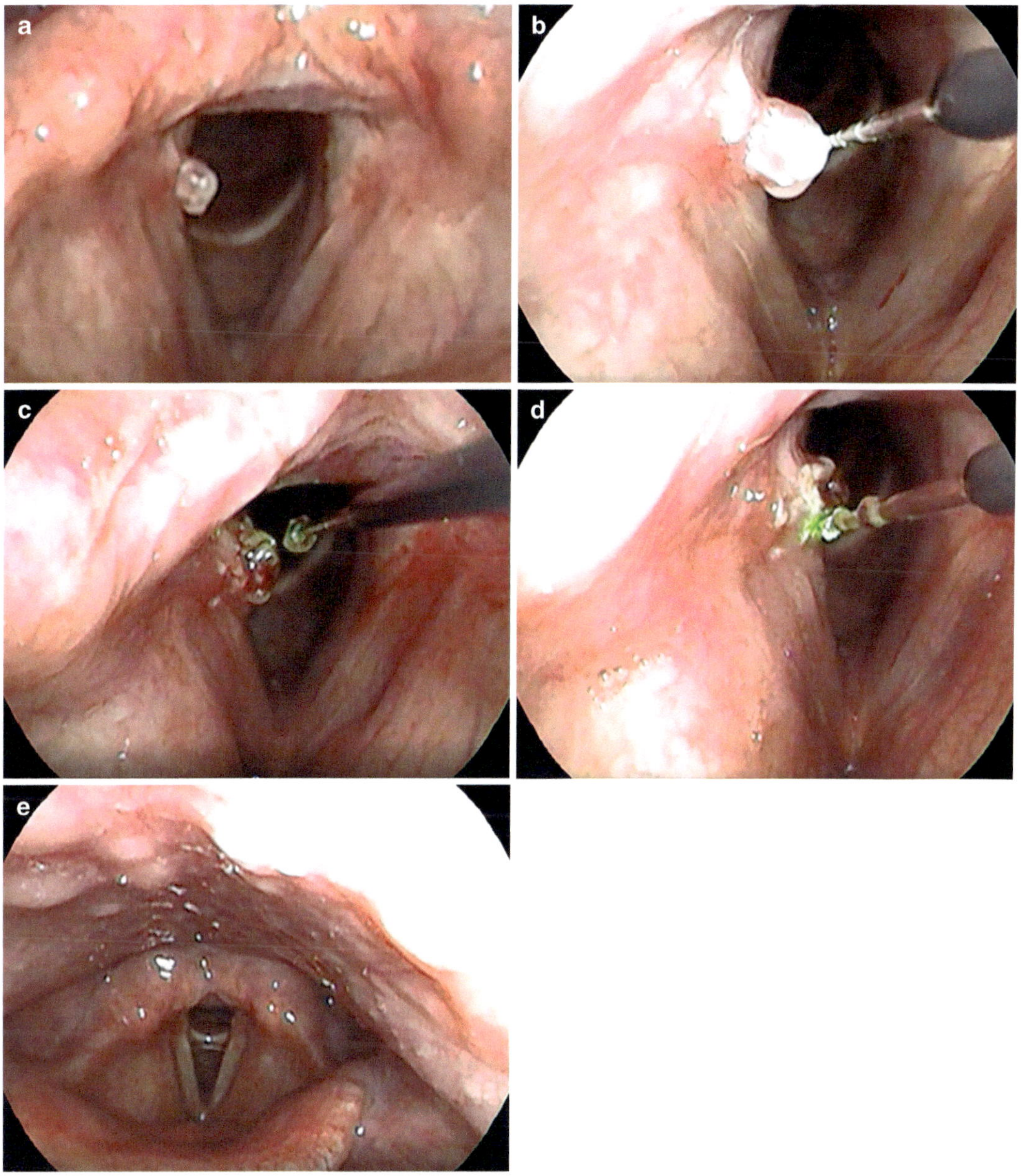

Fig. 7.2 (**a**) A preoperative view of the larynx showing a right vocal process granuloma. (**b**) An endoscopic view of the larynx showing the blue laser glass fiber in contact with the right vocal process granuloma. Note blanching of the lesion during therapy. (**c**) An endoscopic view of the larynx showing the lesion half-way during surgery. (**d**) An endoscopic view of the larynx showing disease regression toward the end of the blue laser therapy. (**e**) Flexible nasopharyngoscopy 3 months after surgery showing complete resolution of the lesion

series of 3 5-FU vocal fold injections to treat vocal fold scar. Due to her glottic insufficiency, she was taken to operating room again for right vocal fold medialization with homograft fascia lata implantation. However, one month postoperatively, the patient's dysphonia recurred. Laryngeal exam showed granuloma formation at the site of implant surgery (Fig. 7.3a). Blue laser was used to vaporize the granuloma (Fig. 7.3b; Video 7.3). Six months following the procedure, the granuloma had disappeared completely (Fig. 7.3c). Medialization remained good.

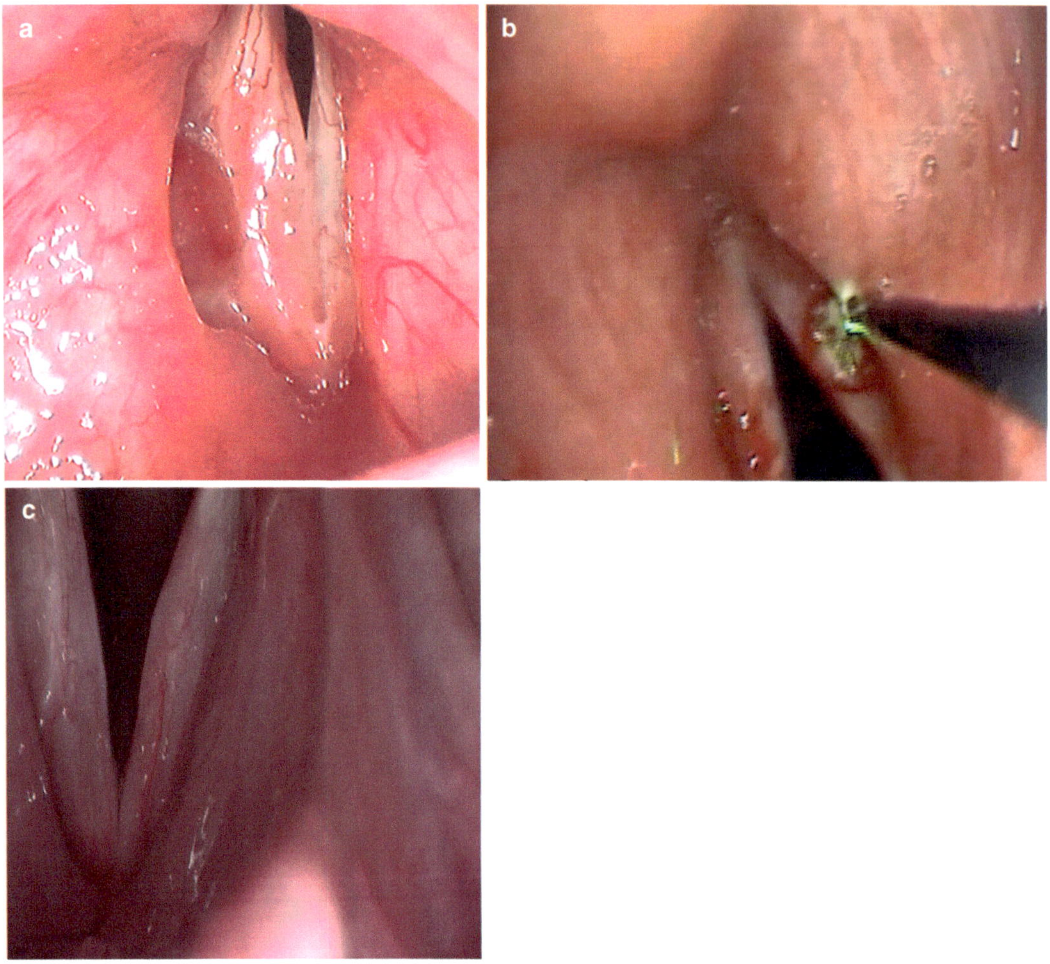

Fig. 7.3 (**a**) The laryngeal examination shows the right vocal fold granuloma. (**b**) In-office blue laser treatment of right vocal fold granuloma was performed using contact and noncontact modes. Settings were 10 watts, 60 ms pulse duration, and 150 ms pulse pause. (**c**) Laryngeal examination 6 months postoperatively showing complete resection of right vocal fold granuloma. Medialization remained good

7.2.4 Case 7.4

This patient was a 68-year-old man with a history of posterior glottic stenosis who presented to our office (RTS) with a posterior left true vocal fold granuloma that had developed as a complication of stent placement.

In-office blue laser treatment was used to vaporize the left posterior vocal fold granuloma (Fig. 7.4a and b). The patient could only tolerate partial ablation in the office, and the patient was taken to the operating room to complete granuloma vaporization. Postoperative examination 6 months after the procedure is shown in Fig. 7.4c.

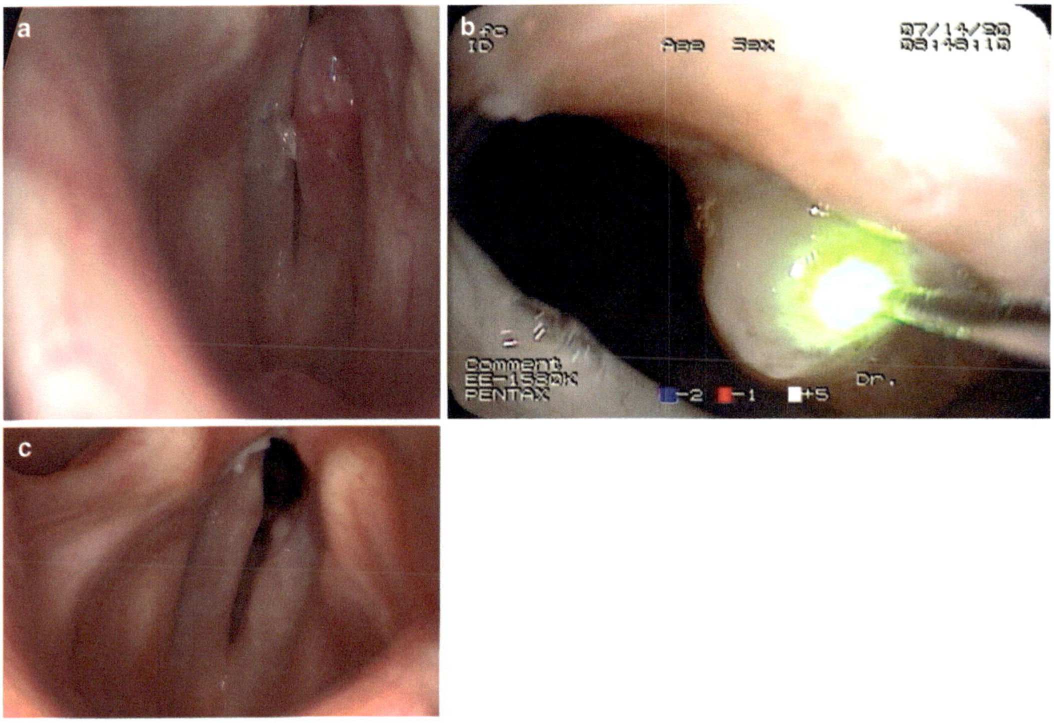

Fig. 7.4 (**a**) Laryngeal examination showing left vocal fold granuloma. (**b**) In-office still image of blue laser treatment of left posterior true vocal fold granuloma. The blue laser fiber was positioned through the working channel of the flexible laryngoscope. Settings were 10 watts, 60 msec pulse duration, and 150 ms pulse pause. Contact and noncontact modes were used. The patient was not able to tolerate the procedure, and it was aborted after partial vaporization of the granuloma and was completed in the operating room. (**c**) Laryngeal examination 6 months after the procedure showing granuloma healing and residual vocal fold deficit related to injury from stent

References

1. Chevalier J. Contact ulcers of the larynx. Ann Otol Rhinol Laryngol. 1982;37(1):227–30.
2. Lee DH, Yoon TM, Lee JK, Lim SC. Surgical treatment outcomes of vocal process granuloma after endotracheal intubation. J Craniofac Surg. 2018;29(4):e387.
3. Shoffel-Havakuk H, Halperin D, Yosef L, Feldberg E, Lahav Y. Lesions of the posterior glottis: clinical and pathologic considerations and treatment outcome. J Voice. 2014;28(263):e1–4.
4. Karkos PD, George M, Van Der Veen J, Atkinson H, Dwivedi RC, et al. Vocal process granulomas: a systematic review of treatment. Ann Otol Rhinol Laryngol. 2014;123(5):314–20.
5. Ylitalo R, Lindestad PA. A retrospective study of contact granuloma. Laryngoscope. 1999;109(3):433–6.
6. Lee SW, Hong HJ, Choi SH, et al. Comparison of treatment modalities for contact granuloma: a nationwide multicenter study. Laryngoscope. 2014;124(5):1187–91.
7. Pham Q, Campbell R, Mattioni J, Sataloff R. Botulinum toxin injections into the lateral cricoarytenoid muscles for vocal process granuloma. J Voice. 2018;32(3):363–6.
8. Hamdan AL, Khalifee E, Jaffal H, Ghanem A. Interarytenoid botulinum toxin a injection for the treatment of vocal process granuloma. J Laryngol Otol. 2019;133(12):1041–5.
9. Wang CT, Lai MS, Lo WC, Liao LJ, Cheng PW. Intralesional steroid injection: an alternative treatment option for vocal process granuloma in ten patients. Clin Otolaryngol. 2013;38(1):77–81.
10. Koufman JA, Rees CJ, Frazier WD, Kilpatrick LA, Wright SC, Halum SL, et al. Office-based laryngeal laser surgery: a review of 443 cases using three wavelengths. Otolaryngol Head Neck Surg. 2007;137(1):146–51.
11. Dominguez LM, Brown RJ, Simpson CB. Treatment outcomes of in-office KTP ablation of vocal fold granulomas. Ann Otol Rhinol Laryngol. 2017;126(12):829–34.

Office-Based Blue Laser Therapy for Recurrent Respiratory Papillomatosis

8

8.1 Introduction

Recurrent respiratory papilloma (RRP) is a disease of the mucosal lining of the respiratory tract caused by the human papilloma virus (HPV). The most common HPV strains identified in RRP of the larynx are the HPV 6 and 11 [1, 2]. Recurrent respiratory papilloma is mostly sexually transmitted, but other modes of transmission also have been described such as hetero inoculation in children [3]. The lesion may be found anywhere in the larynx and may be exophytic, pedunculated, single, or multiple. On histologic examination, the lesion has a finger-like appearance with a central fibrovascular core [4]. Rapid growth may be an ominous sign suggestive of malignant transformation which has been associated with HPV 16 and 18 [5], and other HPV viral types. The main indication for intervention is worsening voice quality and/or shortness of breath secondary to narrowing of the airway. The primary treatment modality of RRP is surgical removal [6–9] although adjunct medical treatments are used as well. In this chapter the authors review several cases of RRP treated in-office using the blue laser.

Supplementary Information The online version contains supplementary material available at https://doi.org/10.1007/978-3-031-71825-0_8.

8.2 Case Presentations

8.2.1 Case 8.1

A 68-year-old male with known recurrent respiratory papillomatosis (RRP) presented to the Voice Clinic (ALH) with dysphonia that had been present for many years duration. The patient had had multiple laryngeal surgeries under general anesthesia for his RRP. On laryngeal examination, he had a lesion occupying more than half the membranous portion of the right vocal fold reaching the vocal process (Fig. 8.1a). Office-based biopsy from the right vocal fold which consisted of two fragments of tan soft tissue measuring in aggregate 0.3 × 0.3 × 0.2 cm was consistent with laryngeal squamous papilloma. The patient underwent office-based blue laser therapy using the 400 micrometers glass fiber. The laser setting was power 10 w, pulse duration 30 ms, and pulse pause 300 ms. The laser was used in contact and near-contact mode (Fig. 8.1b and c; Video 8.1). The procedure was tolerated well by the patient.

8.2.2 Case 8.2

A 43-year-old male presented to the Voice Clinic (ALH) with a chief complaint of dizziness and imbalance. His medical history was positive for reflux disease. Examination of the oral cavity

A. L. Hamdan et al., *Atlas of Office-based Blue Laser Therapy in Laryngology*,
https://doi.org/10.1007/978-3-031-71825-0_8

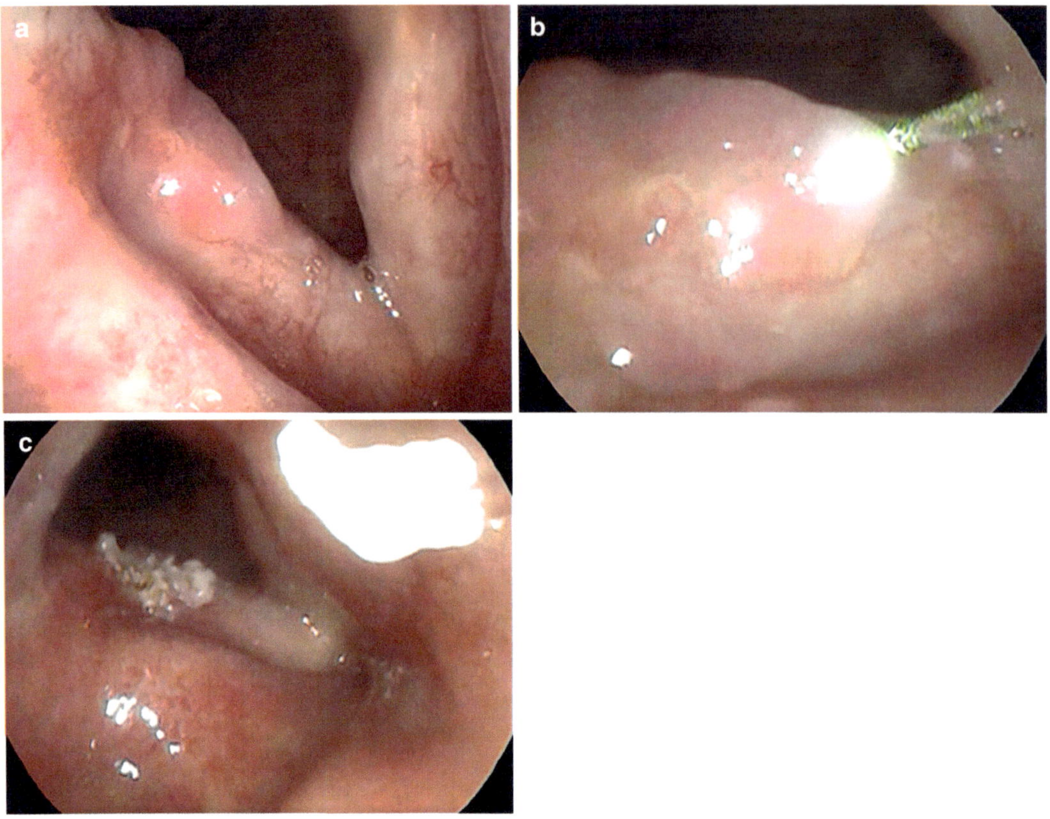

Fig. 8.1 (**a**) An endoscopic view of the larynx showing a lesion occupying more than half the membranous portion of the right vocal fold reaching the vocal process. Note that the appearance of the lesion is not as typical as that of Fig. 8.3a. (**b**) An intraoperative view of the larynx showing the blue laser glass fiber in contact mode against the right vocal fold lesion. (**c**) An image of the larynx toward the end of surgery showing necrotic debris in the surgical bed

revealed a lesion on the anterior pillar of the right tonsil. Nasopharyngeal endoscopy showed a papilloma-like lesion on the laryngeal surface of the epiglottis (Fig. 8.2a). The patient had no voice or swallowing symptoms.

The patient underwent office-based laryngeal biopsy under general anesthesia. Histopathologic examination of the specimen submitted was consistent with squamous papilloma. He subsequently underwent blue laser therapy for his laryngeal lesion using the 400 micrometer glass fiber. Using the flexible fiberoptic nasopharyngoscope, the laser was introduced through the working channel, and a total of 85 Joules was delivered (Fig. 8.2b–d; Video 8.2). The oral lesion also was treated with the blue laser, and a total of 19 Joules was delivered (Fig. 8.2e and f). The procedure was tolerated well by the patient with no complications noted.

8.2.3 Case 8.3

A 30-year-old male presented to the Voice Clinic (ALH) with hoarseness of a few years' duration. The patient had a history of recurrent respiratory papillomatosis that had been treated with several sessions of laser therapy under general anesthesia. The patient denied any history of smoking, voice abuse, allergy, or reflux disease. His Voice Handicap Index-10 (VHI-10) score was 32. Laryngeal endoscopic examination revealed a papillomatous lesion occupying both vocal folds and crossing the anterior commissure (Fig. 8.3a).

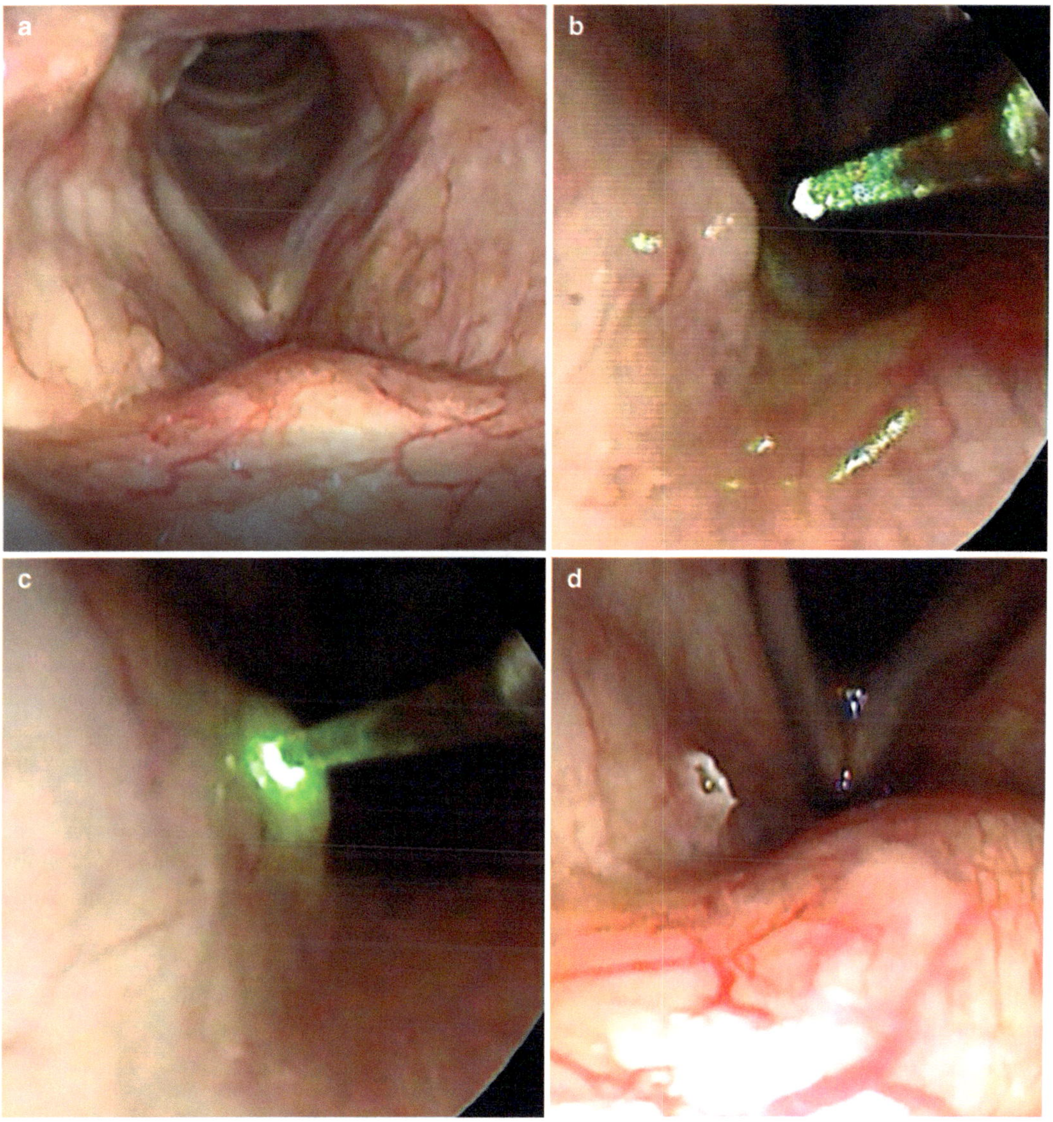

Fig. 8.2 (**a**) An endoscopic view of the larynx showing a papilloma on the laryngeal surface of the epiglottis at the level of the right false vocal fold. Note that the appearance of the lesion is not as typical as that of Fig. 8.3a. (**b**) An endoscopic view of the larynx showing the blue laser in noncontact mode directed toward the lesion. (**c**) An endoscopic view of the larynx showing the blue laser glass fiber in contact with lesion. (**d**) A view of the larynx toward the end of surgery showing complete regression of the lesion. (**e**) A telescopic view of the oral cavity showing a papilloma-like lesion on the surface of the anterior pillar of the right tonsil. (**f**) A telescopic view of the oral cavity showing how the lesion is removed using the blue laser glass fiber. Note the prominent vascularity at the base of the lesion

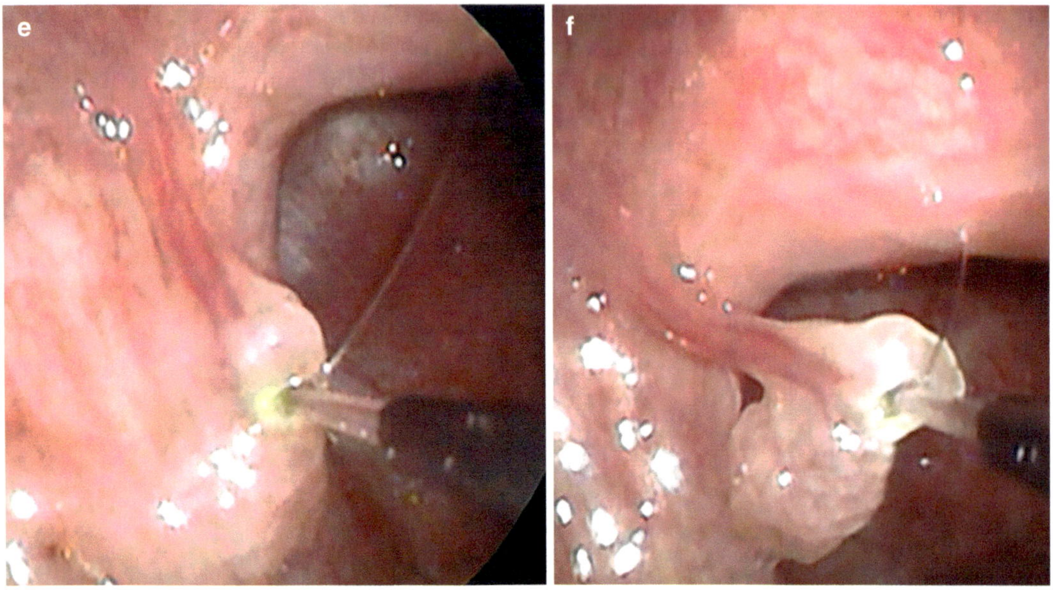

Fig. 8.2 (continued)

The patient underwent office-based blue laser therapy for his laryngeal lesion under local anesthesia. The blue laser was used in contact and noncontact modes, and a total of 200 Joules was delivered (Fig. 8.3b–d; Video 8.3). The procedure was tolerated well by the patient with no complications noted. The patient left the country few days after surgery and was lost to follow-up.

8.2.4 Case 8.4

A 33-year-old male presented to the clinic (ALH) with history of nasal obstruction, itching, and intermittent watery nasal discharge. The patient had no throat symptoms or change in voice quality. On nasal endoscopy he had a septal deviation and bilateral inferior turbinate hypertrophy. Laryngeal examination revealed a papilloma-like lesion over the left aryepiglottic fold. A laryngeal biopsy was taken in-office under local anesthesia (Fig. 8.4a; Video 8.4). The histopathologic examination of the specimen taken (0.2 × 0.1 × 0.1 cm) showed laryngeal squamous papilloma. The patient underwent office-based blue laser therapy for his laryngeal lesion using the contact and noncontact modes (Fig. 8.4b; Video 8.5). The procedure was tolerated well by the patient with no complications noted. On follow-up there was complete regression of the lesion.

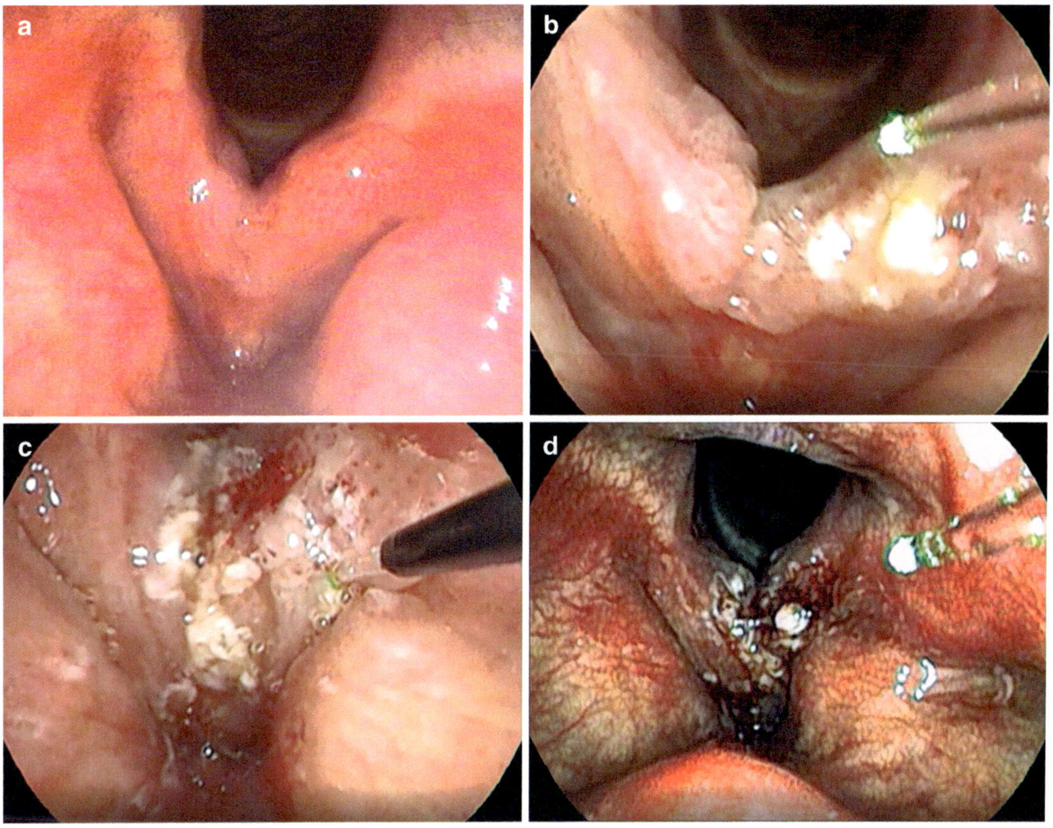

Fig. 8.3 (**a**) An endoscopic view of the larynx showing papillomatous lesions at the glottis involving both vocal folds and crossing the anterior commissure. (**b**) An endoscopic view of the larynx showing the blue laser in non-contact mode. Note blanching of the lesion on the left side. (**c**) An endoscopic view of the larynx showing the blue laser in contact mode against the lesion of the left vocal fold. (**d**) An endoscopic view of the larynx during surgery using the i-scan illumination, which is a digital process technology that enhances the texture and visualization of the mucosal surface blood vessels

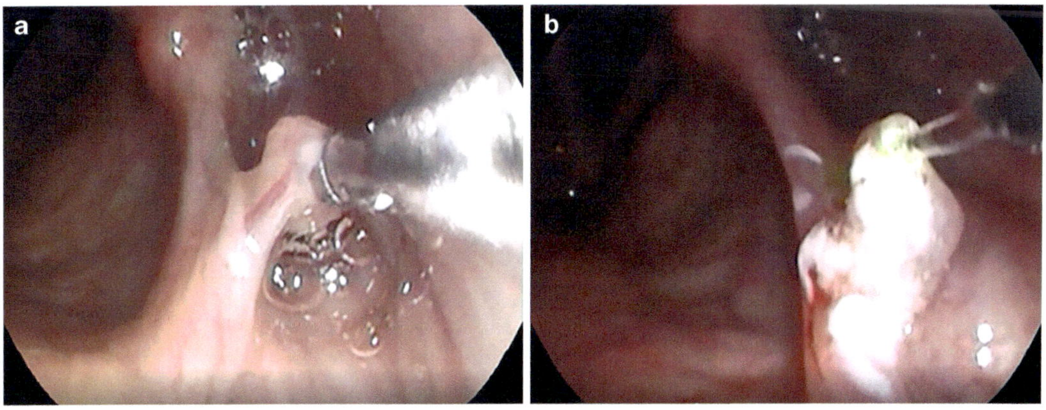

Fig. 8.4 (**a**) An endoscopic view of the larynx showing a biopsy of a papilloma-like lesion at the left aryepiglottic fold. (**b**) An endoscopic view of the larynx showing the blue laser in contact with the lesion

References

1. Bennett RS, Powell KR. Human papillomaviruses: associations between laryngeal papillomas and genital warts. Pediatr Infect Dis J. 1987;6(3):229–32.
2. Weller SC, Stanberry LR. Estimating the population prevalence of HPV. JAMA. 2007;297(8):876–8.
3. Syrjänen S, Puranen M. Human papillomavirus infections in children: the potential role of maternal transmission. Crit Rev Oral Biol Med. 2000;11(2):259–74.
4. Abramson AL, Steinberg BM, Winkler B. Laryngeal papillomatosis: clinical, histopathologic and molecular studies. Laryngoscope. 1987;97(6):678–85.
5. McKaig RG, Baric RS, Olshan AF. Human papillomavirus and head and neck cancer: epidemiology and molecular biology. Head Neck. 1998;20(3):250–65.
6. Zeitels SM, Akst LM, Burns JA, Hillman RE, Broadhurst MS, Anderson RR. Office-based 532-nm pulsed KTP laser treatment of glottal papillomatosis and dysplasia. Ann Otol Rhinol Laryngol. 2006;115(9):679–85.
7. Koufman JA, Rees CJ, Frazier WD, Kilpatrick LA, Wright SC, Halum SL, et al. Office-based laryngeal laser surgery: a review of 443 cases using three wavelengths. Otolaryngol Head Neck Surg. 2007;137(1):146–51.
8. Centric A, Hu A, Heman-Ackah YD, Divi V, Sataloff RT. Office-based pulsed-dye laser surgery for laryngeal lesions: a retrospective review. J Voice. 2014;28(2):262.e9–12.
9. Hamdan AL, Sataloff RT, Ramadan O, Eichorn D, Hawkshaw MJ. Blue laser therapy for recurrent respiratory papillomatosis. In: Hamdan AL, Sataloff RT, Ramadan O, Eichorn D, Hawkshaw MJ, editors. Blue laser surgery in laryngology. Springer Nature; 2023. p. 59–68.

9 Office-Based Blue Laser Therapy for Vocal Fold Leukoplakia

9.1 Introduction

Leukoplakia is a whitish discoloration of the mucosa. When present on the vocal fold, it suggests pathologic changes in the mucosal lining which may be neoplastic [1]. Affected patients can be asymptomatic or can present with dysphonia [2]. Although laryngeal examination using videostroboscopy and narrow band imaging have increased the accuracy of prediction of malignancy in these lesions, a biopsy is needed for definitive diagnosis, particularly when there is a high index of suspicion [3, 4]. Different treatment strategies have been described. These include vocal hygiene therapy [5], surgical excision using microflap technique [6, 7], and laser ablation using various types of lasers the most common of which are the photo-angiolytic lasers which target the submucosal microvasculature of the lesion [8–13]. Photo-angiolytic lasers can be used in the operating room or in-office. A single or multiple sessions may be needed to achieve complete regression of the lesion.

Supplementary Information The online version contains supplementary material available at https://doi.org/10.1007/978-3-031-71825-0_9.

9.2 Case Presentations

9.2.1 Case 9.1

A 35-year-old male heavy smoker presented to the Voice Clinic (ALH) with hoarseness of a few years' duration. The patient had a history of reflux disease but had no history of voice abuse or allergy. His Voice Handicap Index (VHI-10) score was 2. Acoustic analysis showed a fundamental frequency (F0) of 92.81 Hz, habitual pitch of 100.38 Hz, jitter 0.67, shimmer 2.49, a noise-to-harmonic ratio (NHR) of 0.123, and a voice turbulence index (VTI) of 0.051. Aerodynamic analysis showed a maximum phonation time (MPT) of 29.61 seconds. Laryngeal endoscopic examination revealed bilateral vocal fold leukoplakia (Fig. 9.1a). Vocal fold biopsies were taken in-office under local anesthesia, and the pathologic examination showed mild reactive atypia but no malignancy. The patient underwent two sessions of office-based blue laser therapy. The setting used was power 10 W, pulse duration 30 ms, pulse pause 300 ms (Fig. 9.1b; Video 9.1). The procedures were tolerated well by the patient with no complications noted.

On follow-up 2 months later, the patient had marked improvement in his voice quality. His VHI-10 score dropped to 0. Acoustic analysis showed an increase in the F0 to 105.8 Hz. Laryngeal examination revealed 90% regression of the lesion (Fig. 9.1c).

A. L. Hamdan et al., *Atlas of Office-based Blue Laser Therapy in Laryngology*,
https://doi.org/10.1007/978-3-031-71825-0_9

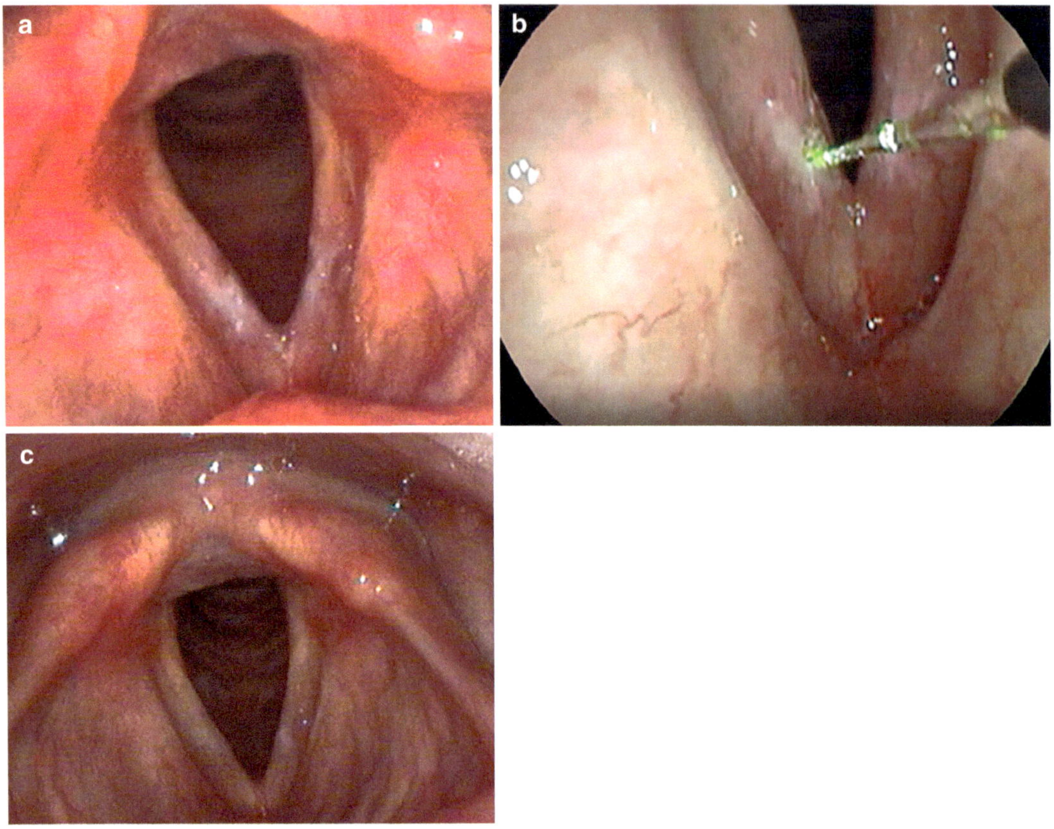

Fig. 9.1 (**a**) An endoscopic view of the larynx showing bilateral vocal fold leukoplakia at the anterior and mid-membranous portions of the vocal folds. (**b**) Intra-operative view of the larynx showing the blue laser glass fiber in contact with the right vocal fold leukoplakia. (**c**) A post-operative view of the larynx 2 months later showing almost complete regression of the lesion of the right vocal fold, and partial regression of the lesion of the left vocal fold

9.2.2 Case 9.2

A 63-year-old male presented to the Voice Clinic (ALH) with hoarseness associated with intermittent dyspnea and stridor. The patient denied any history of phonotrauma, allergy or reflux disease. His Voice Handicap Index-10 (VHI-10) on presentation was 10. Acoustic analysis showed a fundamental frequency (F0) of 123.22 Hz, habitual pitch (HP) of 109.96 Hz, jitter 1.7, shimmer 5, a noise-to-harmonics ration (NHR) of 0.17, and a voice turbulence index (VTI) of 0.79. Aerodynamic parameters showed a maximum phonation time (MPT) of 8.17 seconds. Laryngeal flexible endoscopic examination revealed a right vocal fold leukoplakia (Fig. 9.2a).

The patient underwent office-based biopsy of the lesion under local anesthesia (Fig. 9.2b). Histologic examination revealed no malignancy. The patient underwent in-office-based blue laser therapy for his right vocal fold lesion using contact and non-contact modes. A total of 117 Joules was delivered. The procedure was tolerated well by the patient with no complications noted. On follow up 6 weeks later, he had complete regression of the lesion (Fig. 9.2c and d).

9.2.3 Case 9.3

A 70-year-old male heavy smoker presented to the Voice Clinic (ALH) with hoarseness of a few years' duration. The patient denied any history of phonotrauma, reflux disease or allergy. His Voice Handicap Index −10 (VHI-10) score was 28. Laryngeal flexible endoscopic examination revealed bilateral vocal fold leukoplakia (Fig. 9.3a). The patient underwent office-based

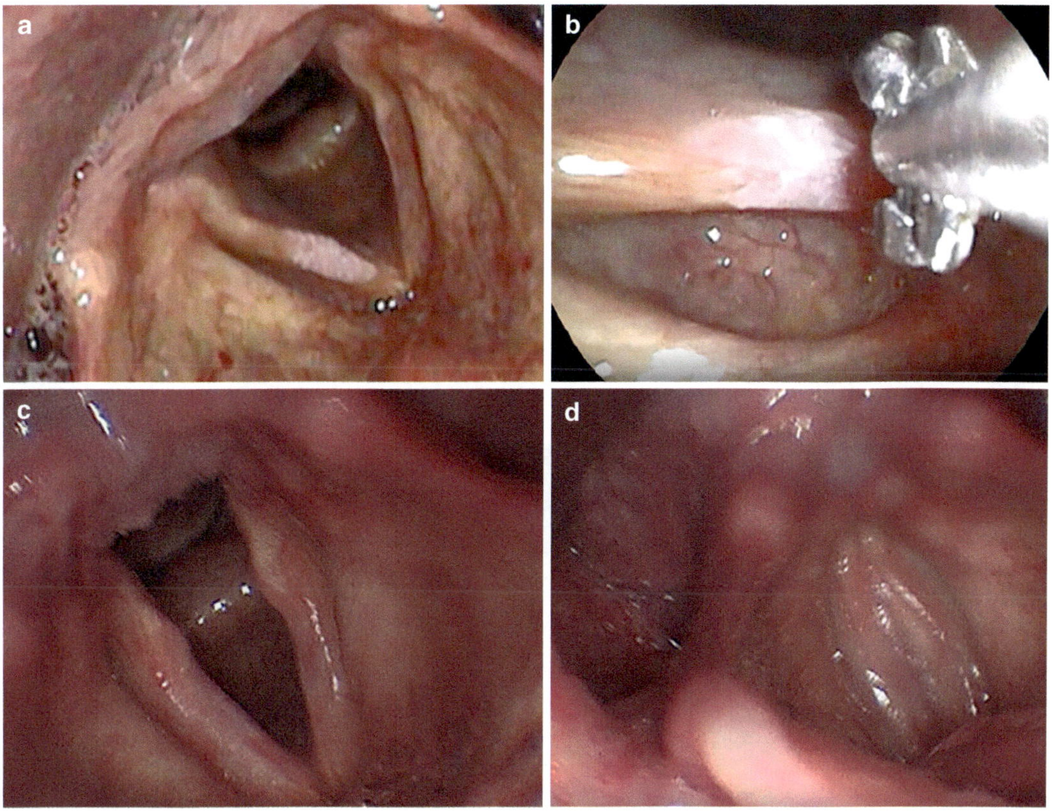

Fig. 9.2 (**a**) A pre-operative view of the larynx showing a right vocal fold leukoplakia. (**b**) An endoscopic view of the larynx showing the cup forceps directed toward the lesion. (**c**) An endoscopic view of the larynx 6 weeks after surgery showing complete regression of the lesion. (**d**) An endoscopic view of the larynx 6 weeks after surgery showing complete closure of the vocal folds during phonation

biopsy of both lesions under local anesthesia (Fig. 9.3b). Histopathologic examination showed low-grade squamous dysplasia of the left vocal fold and high-grade squamous dysplasia of the right vocal fold. The patient underwent blue laser therapy for his vocal fold lesions under local anesthesia using power 10 watts, pulse duration 30 ms, and pulse pause 300 ms (Fig. 9.3c and d). A total of 298 J was delivered during the procedure. The laser was used in contact and non-contact modes. The procedure was tolerated well by the patient with no complications noted.

On follow-up 4 weeks later, the patient presented with improvement in his voice quality. His VHI-10 score dropped to 7. Laryngeal endoscopic examination showed partial regression of the lesion bilaterally. The patient underwent another office-based blue laser therapy session for the treatment of his lesion following which he had further decrease in his VHI-10 which dropped to 4. Laryngeal endoscopic examination 5 months later showed almost complete resolution of the lesion except for mild residual disease on the medial surface of the left vocal fold process and mild disease on the lower lip of the right vocal fold (mid-membranous portion) (Fig. 9.3e).

9.2.4 Case 9.4

A 51-year-old male heavy smoker presented to the Voice Clinic (ALH) with hoarseness of 2 weeks duration. The patient denied any history of phonotrauma, reflux disease, or allergy. His Voice Handicap Index −10 (VHI-10) score was 18. On laryngeal examination, he had right vocal fold leukoplakia, which has a biofilm-like appear-

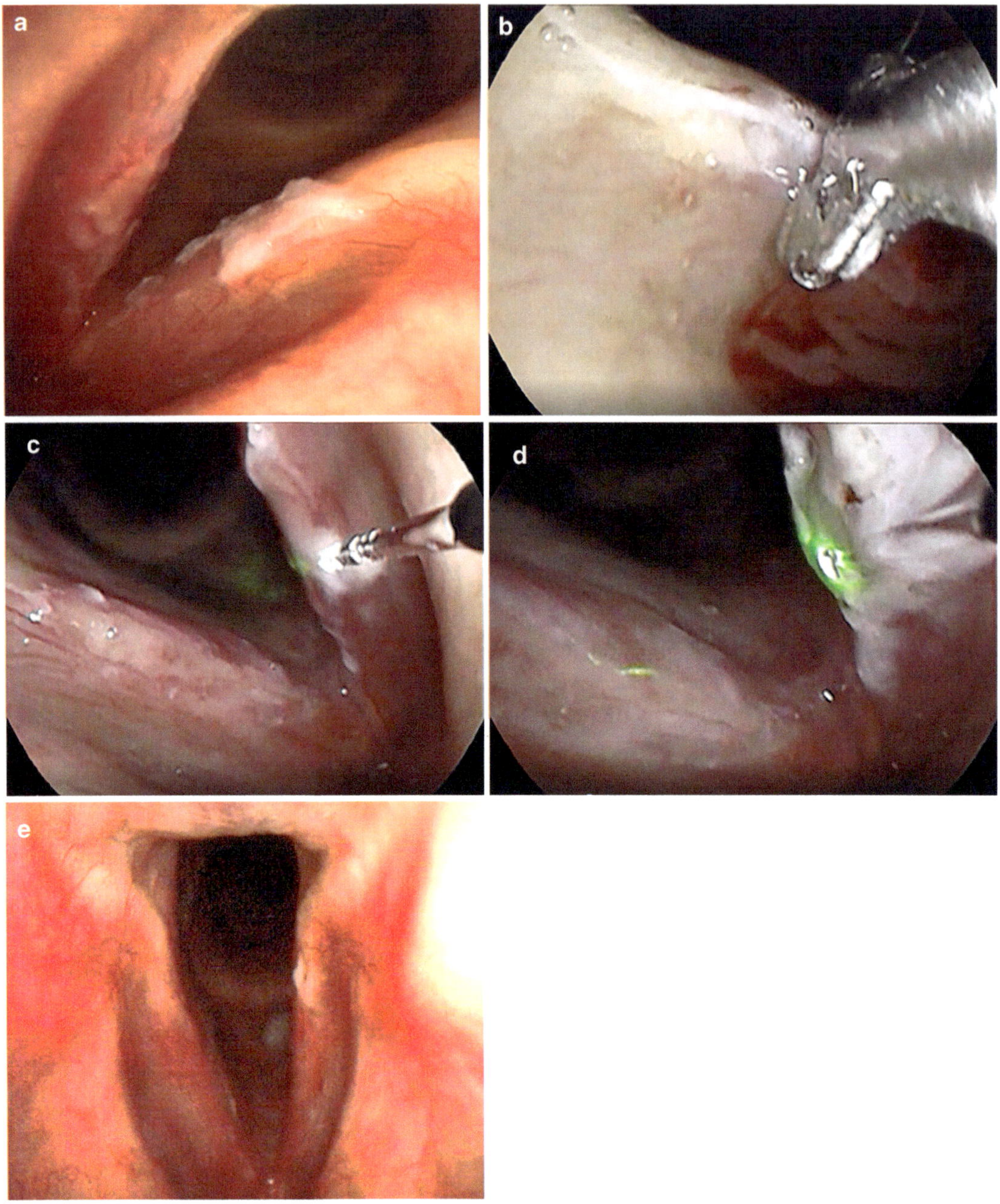

Fig. 9.3 (**a**) Pre-operative view of the larynx showing bilateral vocal fold lesions. (**b**) Endoscopic view showing the cup forceps directed toward the lesion. (**c**) Intra-operative view showing the blue laser targeting the lesion on the left vocal fold. (**d**) Intra-operative view showing the blue laser glass fiber in contact with the lower lip of the left vocal fold. (**e**) Post-operative view of the larynx 5 months after surgery showing almost complete disease regression. Note mild residual disease on the medial surface of the left vocal process, and mild residual disease on the mid-third of the right vocal fold (lower lip)

ance, and a reactive lesion on the left vocal fold (Fig. 9.4a). The patient was treated with antibiotics (levofloxacin 750 mg/day and anti-fungal (Fluconazole 100 mg/day) medications for 6 weeks to no avail. On follow up he had no improvement in voice quality and no interval change on laryngeal examination. The patient underwent office-based biopsy of both vocal

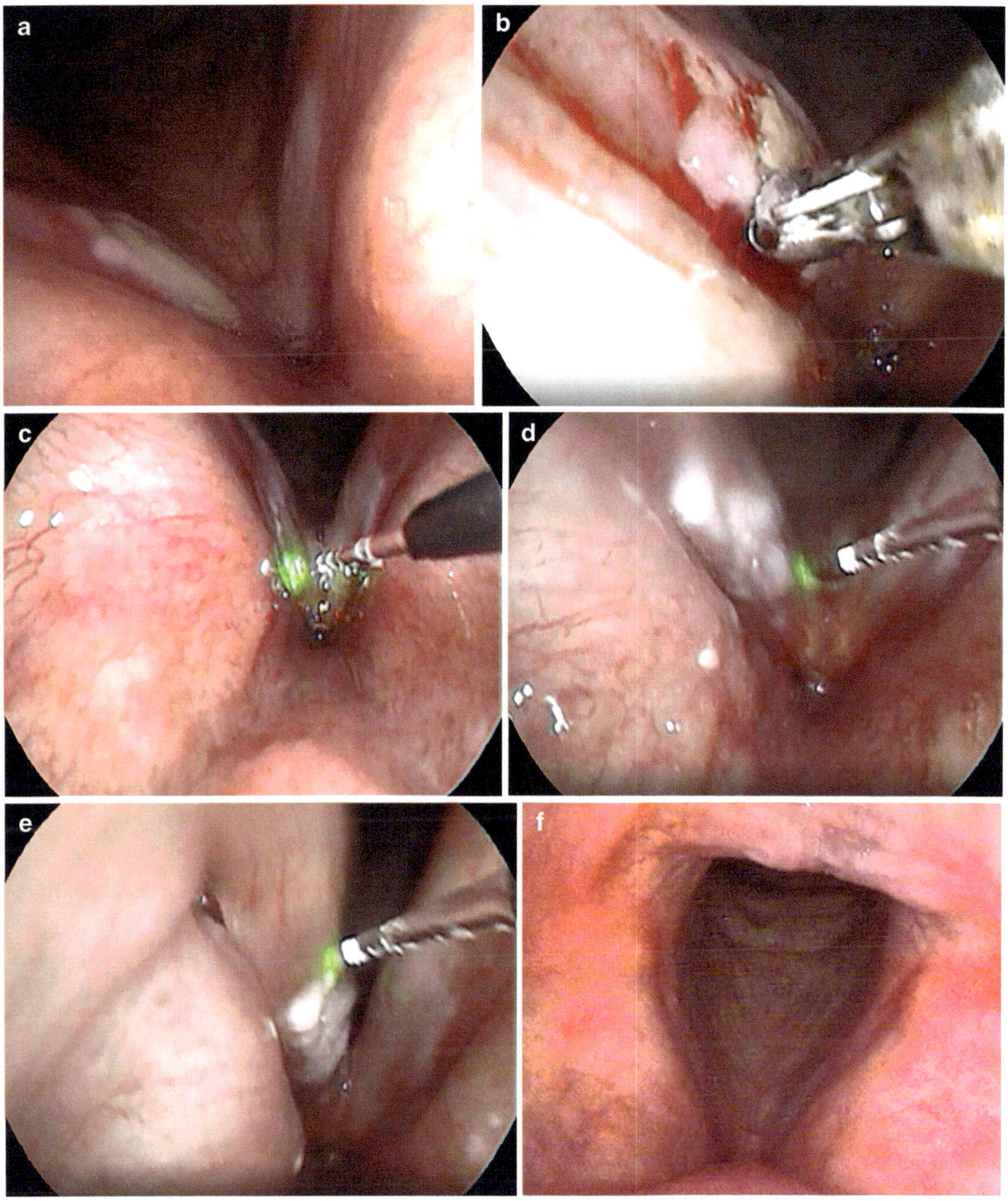

Fig. 9.4 (**a**) Pre-operative view showing right vocal fold biofilm-like appearance. Note reactive changes in the mucosal lining of the left vocal fold. (**b**) Intra-op view showing a biopsy of the right vocal fold lesion. (**c**) An intra-operative view of the larynx showing the blue laser in non-contact mode. (**d**) An intra-operative view showing blanching of the lesion of the right vocal fold following blue laser therapy. (**e**) Intra-operative view showing blue laser in contact mode against the posterior edge of the lesion of the right vocal fold. (**f**) A post-operative view 6 weeks after surgery showing complete resolution of the lesion

folds which revealed mild dysplasia bilaterally (Fig. 9.4b).

The patient underwent office-based blue laser therapy for his vocal fold lesions under local anesthesia using power 10 watts, pulse duration 30 ms and pulse pause 300 ms. A total of 82 J was delivered during the procedure. The laser was used in contact and non-contact mode).

Figure 9.4c–e; Video 9.2). The procedure was tolerated well by the patient with no complications noted. On follow-up 6 weeks later, the patient had marked improvement in his voice quality. His VHI-10 score dropped to 4. Laryngeal endoscopic examination showed complete resolution of the lesion on the right vocal fold (Fig. 9.4f).

9.2.5 Case 9.5

A 44-year-old male smoker presented to the Voice Clinic (ALH) with hoarseness and loss of range that had been present few months. The patient had **a** history of voice overuse and abuse. He denied any history of allergy or reflux disease. His Voice Handicap Index-10 score (VHI-10) was 25. Flexible endoscopic laryngeal examination revealed a right vocal fold leukoplakia with diffuse inflammation of the vocal fold (Fig. 9.5a).

The patient underwent office-based biopsy of the right vocal fold under local anesthesia (Fig. 9.5b). Histopathologic examination revealed no malignancy. Subsequently, the patient underwent office-based blue laser therapy for his right vocal fold leukoplakia using the non-contact mode (Fig. 9.5c and d). A total of 53 Joules was delivered. The procedure was tolerated well by the patient with no complications noted.

9.2.6 Case 9.6

This 96-year-old male with a history of laryngopharyngeal reflux, coronary artery disease, and

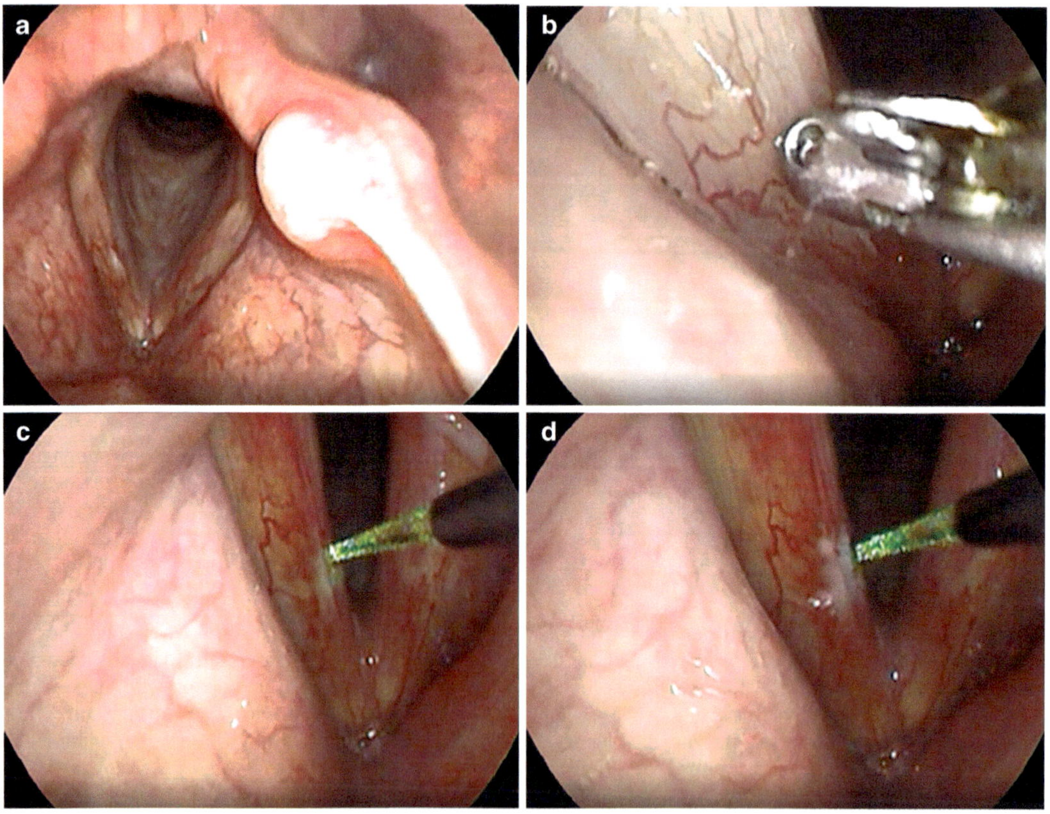

Fig. 9.5 (**a**) An endoscopic view of the larynx showing right vocal fold leukoplakia. (**b**) A view of the larynx showing biopsy of the right vocal fold lesion. (**c**) An endoscopic view of the larynx showing the blue laser in non-contact mode. (**d**) An endoscopic view of the larynx toward the end of blue laser therapy showing blanching of the lesion

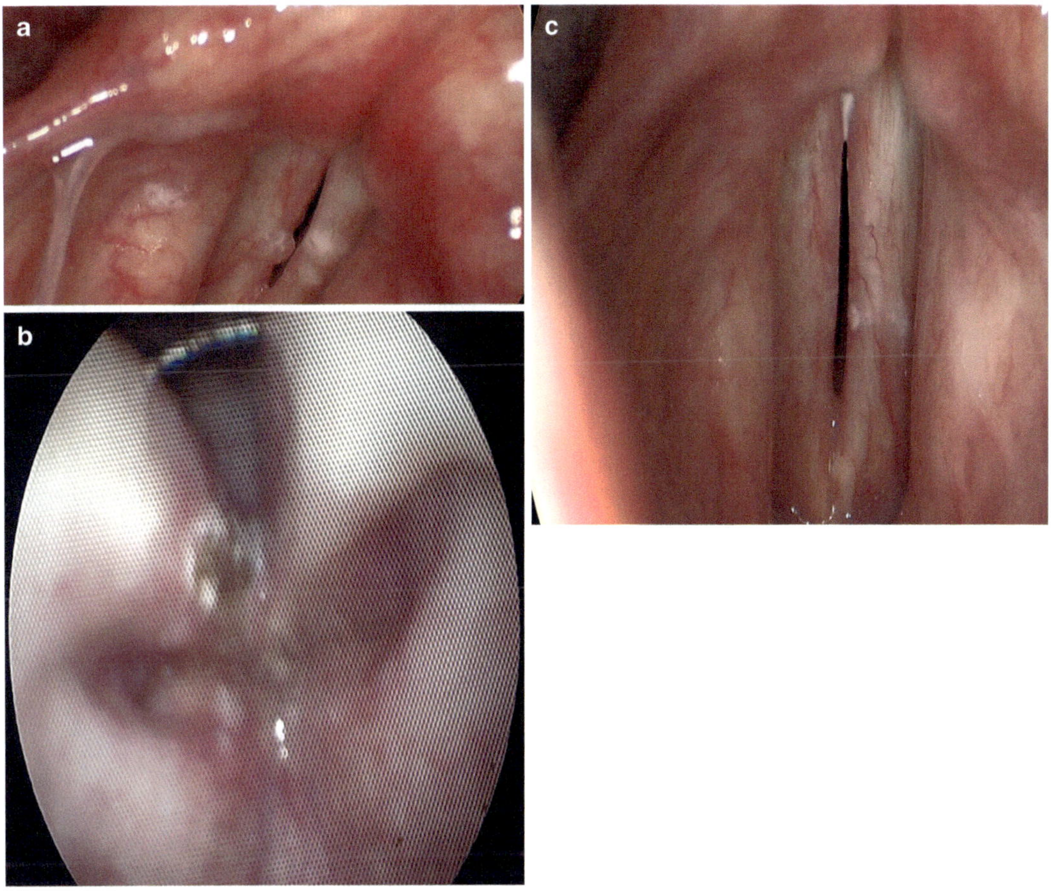

Fig. 9.6 (**a**) Laryngeal examination showing right vocal fold leukoplakia and mass, and superficial left vocal fold leukoplakia. (**b**) In office blue laser ablation of right vocal fold leukoplakia was performed in contact mode with settings of 6 watts, 60 ms pulse duration, 300 ms pulse pause. (**c**) Laryngeal examination showing partial regression of left vocal fold reactive mass and complete right mass regression and leukoplakia healing 4 months after the procedure. The vocal fold was no stiffer than it had been prior to blue laser therapy

atrial fibrillation presented to our office (RTS) with dysphonia related primarily to recurrent, multiple leukoplakia (Fig. 9.6a). The patient had undergone numerous laryngeal procedures including bilateral thyroplasty, fat injection of the right vocal fold, and previous biopsies of leukoplakia that had shown no malignancy. Due to his heart condition, the decision was made to perform in-office leukoplakia vaporization with blue laser (Fig. 9.6b). Four months later, the right vocal fold leukoplakia has healed totally (Fig. 9.6c).

References

1. Kramer IR, Lucas RB, Pindborg JJ, Sobin LH. Definition of leukoplakia and related lesions: an aid to studies on oral precancer. Oral Surg Oral Med Oral Pathol. 1978;46(4):518–39.
2. Gailey MP, Hoffman H. Leukoplakia. In: Sataloff RT, editor. Sataloff's comprehensive textbook of otolaryngology head & neck surgery (laryngology). JP Medical Ltd; 2016. p. 901–14.
3. Isenberg JS, Crozier DL, Dailey SH. Institutional and comprehensive review of laryngeal leukoplakia. Ann Otol Rhinol Laryngol. 2008;117(1):74–9.

4. Chen M, Li C, Yang Y, Cheng L, Wu H. A morphological classification for vocal fold leukoplakia. Braz J Otorhinolaryngol. 2019;85(5):588–96.
5. Gao XW, Huang YW, Liu LY, Ouyang J. Use videostrobokymography to quantitatively analyze the vibratory characteristics before and after conservative medical treatment of vocal fold leukoplakia. J Voice. 2016;30(2):215–20.
6. Gale N, Michaels L, Luzar B, Poljak M, Zidar N, Fischinger J, et al. Current review on squamous intraepithelial lesions of the larynx. Histopathology. 2009;54(6):639–56.
7. Schweinfurth JM, Powitzky E, Ossoff RH. Regression of laryngeal dysplasia after serial microflap excision. Ann Otol Rhinol Laryngol. 2001;110(9):811–4.
8. Zeitels SM, Akst LM, Burns JA, Hillman RE, Broadhurst MS, Anderson RR. Office-based 532-nm pulsed KTP laser treatment of glottal papillomatosis and dysplasia. Ann Otol Rhinol Laryngol. 2006;115(9):679–85.
9. Rees CJ, Halum SL, Wijewickrama RC, Koufman JA, Postma GN. Patient tolerance of in-office pulsed dye laser treatments to the upper aerodigestive tract. Otolaryngol Head Neck Surg. 2006;134(6):1023–7.
10. Koufman JA, Rees CJ, Frazier WD, Kilpatrick LA, Wright SC, Halum SL, et al. Office-based laryngeal laser surgery: a review of 443 cases using three wavelengths. Otolaryngol Head Neck Surg. 2007;137(1):146–51.
11. Mouadeb DA, Belafsky PC. In-office laryngeal surgery with the 585nm pulsed dye laser (PDL). Otolaryngol Head Neck Surg. 2007;137(3):477–81.
12. Koss SL, Baxter P, Panossian H, Woo P, Pitman MJ. Serial in-office laser treatment of vocal fold leukoplakia: disease control and voice outcomes. Laryngoscope. 2017;127(7):1644–51.
13. Hamdan AL, Ghanem A, Abou Raji Feghali P, Hosri J, Abi Zeid Daou C, Abou-Rizk S. Office-based blue laser therapy for vocal fold leukoplakia: a preliminary report of 12 cases. OTO Open. 2023;7(2):e59.

Rare Applications of Office-Based Blue Laser Therapy

10

10.1 Introduction

The blue laser is a hybrid laser with dual properties, cutting and photo-angiolysis. Its effect on tissue is determined mostly by the distance to target, divergence of the laser beam, and duration of exposure [1]. Its application in laryngology is not limited to the treatment of benign and premalignant structural abnormalities of the vocal folds [2]. This chapter describes rare application of the blue laser in an office-setting.

10.2 Case Presentation

10.2.1 Case 10.1

A 71-year-old female, heavy smoker, presented to the voice clinic (ALH) with a history of thyroidectomy performed five years prior to our evaluation following which she developed stridor that necessitated a tracheotomy. Several attempts at decannulation had been made with no success. Laryngeal examination revealed bilateral vocal fold paralysis with a glottal gap of 1–2 mm. Glottal widening procedures were discussed with the patient, and she elected to undergo office-based blue laser cordectomy (Fig. 10.1a and b; Video 10.1). The blue laser glass fiber (400 micrometer) was used in contact and noncontact modes (power 10, pulse duration 10 ms, and pulse pause 150 ms). The procedure was tolerated well by the patient with no complications. On follow-up six weeks later, laryngeal examination showed widening of the glottal gap to 6–7 mm. Twelve weeks later, the patient was decannulated successfully. During her last follow-up visit 5 months after laser laryngeal surgery, the patient was doing well with no shortness of breath. Her Dyspnea Severity Index (DSI) score was 3, and her Voice Handicap Index-10 (VHI-10) score was 2.

10.2.2 Case 10.2

A 47-year-old female smoker presented to the clinic (ALH) with recurrent throat symptoms. The patient denied any history of allergy or reflux disease. Endoscopic examination revealed a papilloma-like lesion at the base of the tongue on the left side (Fig. 10.2a). The patient underwent office-based blue laser therapy under local anesthesia. The blue laser was used in contact and noncontact modes (Fig. 10.2b–d). The laser setting was power 10 watts, pulse duration 30 ms, and pulse pause 300 ms. The procedure was tolerated well by the patient with no complications noted. On follow-up four months

Supplementary Information The online version contains supplementary material available at https://doi.org/10.1007/978-3-031-71825-0_10.

A. L. Hamdan et al., *Atlas of Office-based Blue Laser Therapy in Laryngology*,
https://doi.org/10.1007/978-3-031-71825-0_10

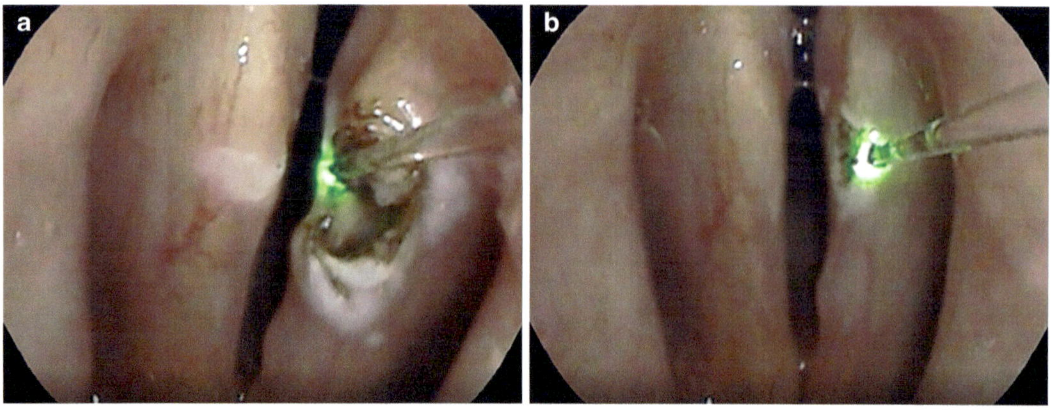

Fig. 10.1 (**a**) An endoscopic view of the larynx showing the blue laser in contact mode at the tip of the left vocal process. (**b**) An endoscopic view of the larynx showing the blue laser cutting the medial and inferior surface of the vocal fold

later, endoscopic examination revealed complete regression of the lesion (Fig. 10.2e).

10.2.3 Case 10.3

This 57-year-old man presented to our practice (RTS) with subglottic stenosis after prolonged intubation following thyroidectomy. He was taken to the operating room for laryngotracheal resection and dilation. However, 3 weeks after that procedure, he presented with anterior subglottic polypoid inflammatory changes. The patient had in-office blue laser treatment for subglottic stenosis (Fig. 10.3a and b; Video 10.2). He did not appear for follow up.

10.2.4 Case 10.4

A 32-year-old female with LPR presented to the office (RTS) with dysphonia despite having had multiple voice therapy sessions and multiple laryngeal procedures. Her dysphonia was related primarily to glottic insufficiency and bilateral vocal fold scar. She was taken to operating room for homograft fascia lata implantation and 5 FU vocal fold injection. 2 weeks later, she presented to the office with partially extruded fascia (Fig. 10.4a.) The blue laser was used to vaporize the extruded fascia without disturbing the fascia that remained in good condition (Fig. 10.4b). Six months after the procedure, the extruded fascia completely disappeared (Fig. 10.4c).

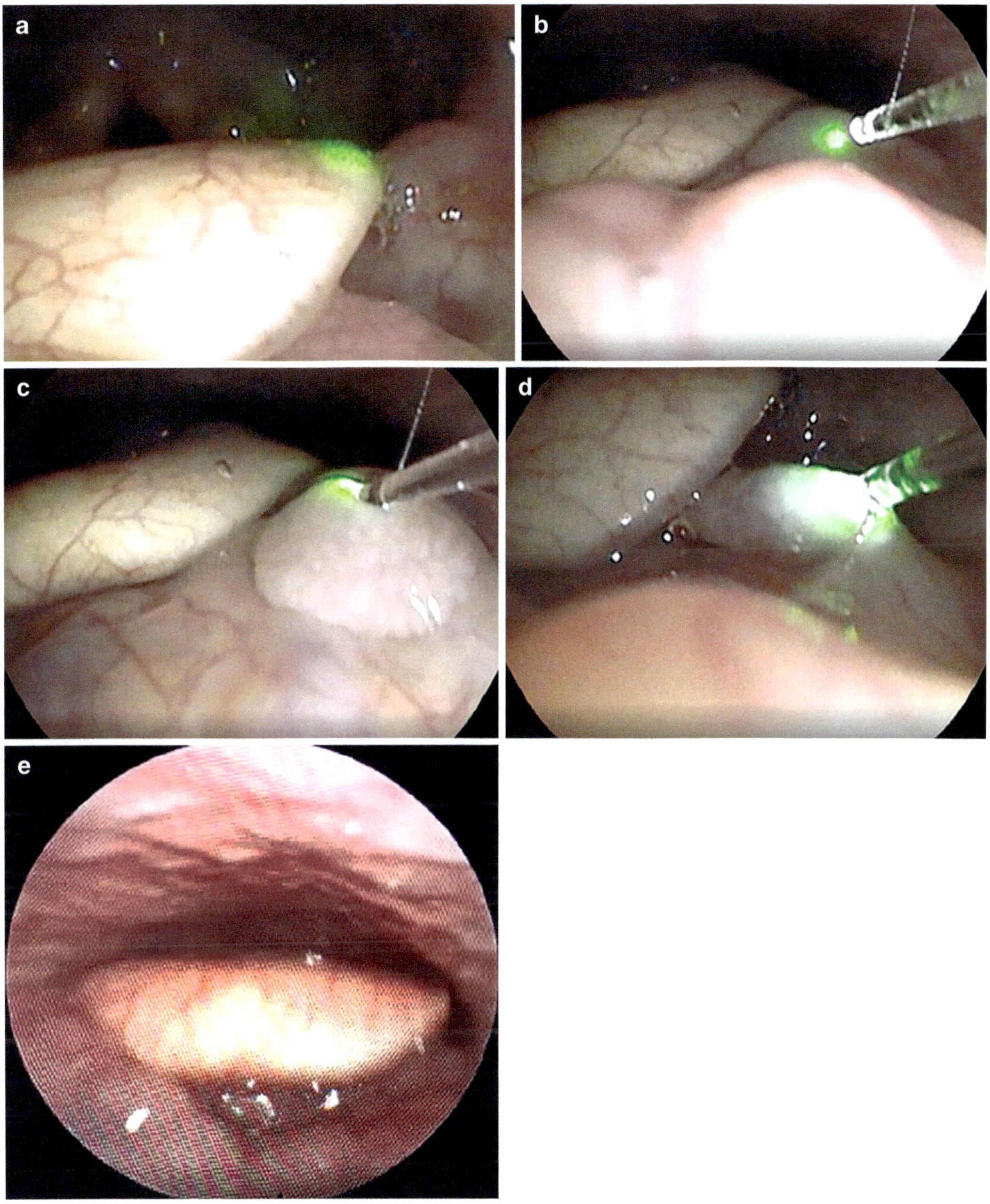

Fig. 10.2 (**a**) An endoscopic view showing the papilloma-like lesion at the base of the tongue. (**b**) An endoscopic view of the base of tongue showing the blue laser in non-contact mode near the lesion. (**c**) An endoscopic view of the base of tongue showing the blue laser in contact mode against the lesion. (**d**) An endoscopic view of the base of tongue showing blanching of the lesion during surgery. (**e**) An endoscopic view of the base of tongue showing complete regression of the lesion

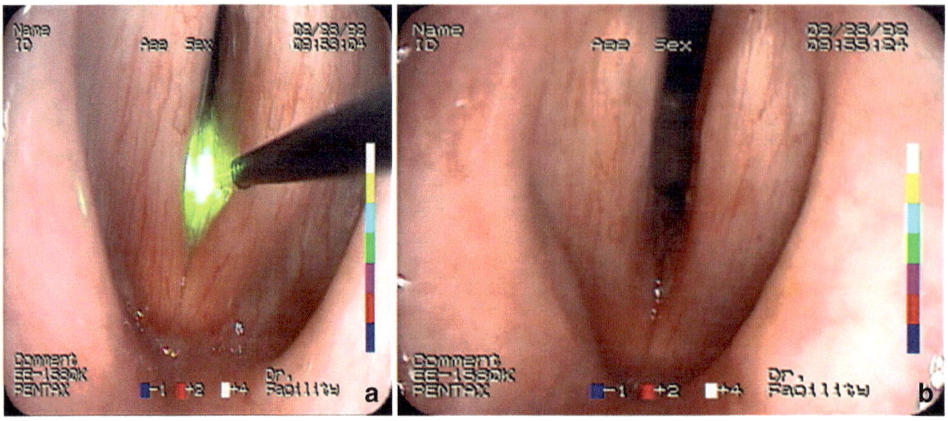

Fig. 10.3 (**a**) Still image taken during beginning of in-office blue laser vaporization of subglottic polypoid inflammation. Contact and noncontact modes were used at 10 watts, 60 ms pulse duration, and 150 ms pulse pause. (**b**) Still image taken immediately after in-office blue laser vaporization of subglottic stenosis

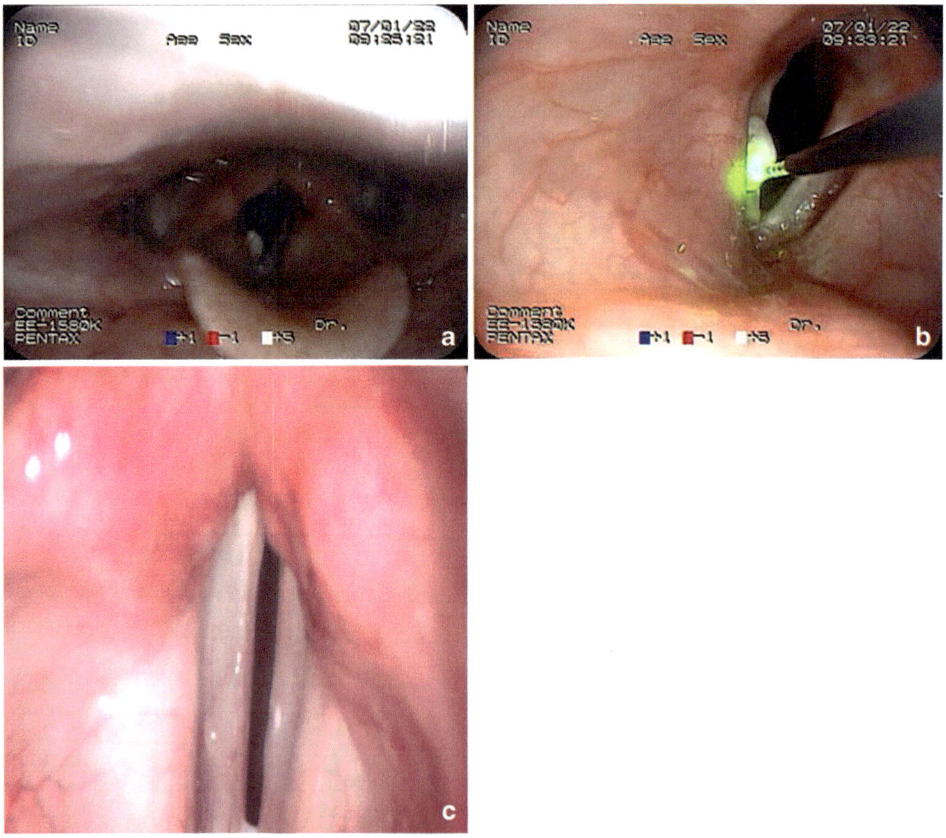

Fig. 10.4 (**a**) Laryngeal examination showing right partial fascia extrusion. (**b**) In-office blue laser vaporization of right vocal fold partial fascia extrusion using contact mode and setting of 10 watts, 60 ms pulse duration, and 150 ms pulse pause. Only the extruded portion of fascia was treated. The retained portion in good position was not disturbed. (**c**) Laryngeal examination 6 months after the procedure showing complete vocal fold healing. Glottic closure and voice were better than they had been prior to fascia implantation, but not perfect

References

1. Hess MM, Fleischer S, Ernstberger M. New 445 nm blue laser for laryngeal surgery combines photoangiolytic and cutting properties. Eur Arch Otorrinolaringol. 2018;275(6):1557–67.
2. Hamdan AL, Sataloff RT, Ramadan O, Eichorn D, Hawkshaw MJ. Blue laser surgery in laryngology. Springer Nature; 2023.

Index

A

Acoustic analysis, 8, 12, 13, 23–25, 31, 32, 34–36, 40–42, 69, 70
Acoustic and aerodynamic analysis, 42
Aerodynamic analysis, 23, 42

B

Bilateral thyroplasty, 75
Bilateral vocal fold leukoplakia, 70
Blue laser, 1, 59, 77
Blue laser glass fiber, 77
Bradycardia, 4

C

Carbon dioxide (CO_2) laser, 1
Conservative therapy, 57
COVID-19 infection, 7

D

Dexamethasone, 16, 23, 52
Dysphonia, 54
Dyspnea Severity Index (DSI), 23, 25, 32, 34, 77

E

Epidermoid cysts, 39

G

General anesthesia, 64–65
Glottic insufficiency, 54

H

Human papilloma virus (HPV), 63
Hypotension, 4

I

Intensive reflux management, 57

L

Laryngeal examination, 40, 42, 43, 45, 49–52, 69, 71, 77
Laryngeal flexible endoscopy, 9
Laryngeal squamous papilloma, 66
Laryngeal videostroboscopy, 42, 49
Laryngopharyngeal reflux (LPR), 54, 57, 58
Laser therapy, 16, 52
Local anesthesia, 4, 10, 66, 69, 71, 73, 77

M

Maximum phonation time (MPT), 7
Microflap technique, 23

N

Nasal endoscopy, 66
Nasopharyngeal endoscopy, 64
Noise-to-harmonics ratio (NHR), 16

O

Office-based blue laser therapy, 2, 7–10, 12–14, 16, 36, 39, 40, 42, 43, 52, 53, 58, 63, 66, 74, 77
Office-based laryngeal biopsy, 64
Office-based laryngeal surgery, 3
Office-based laser therapy, 7, 23, 39

P

Papillary thyroid carcinoma, 58
Phonomicrosurgery, 23
Phonotrauma, 49, 70, 71
Post-operative acoustic analysis, 30
Potassium titanyl phosphate (KTP) laser, 1
Pulse dye laser (PDL), 1

R

Recurrent respiratory papillomatosis (RRP), 63
Reinke's edema (RE), 23, 25–33, 35–37
Residual submucosal hematoma, 54

A. L. Hamdan et al., *Atlas of Office-based Blue Laser Therapy in Laryngology*,
https://doi.org/10.1007/978-3-031-71825-0

S
Small particles, 4
Squamous papilloma, 64
Stridor, 77
Subglottic stenosis, 78
Submucosal hemorrhage, 10

T
Thulium laser, 1
Topical anesthesia, 3, 4

V
Vocal fold biopsies, 69
Vocal fold cysts, 39
Vocal fold granuloma, 57
Vocal fold paralysis, 77
Vocal fold polyps, 7
Vocal fold varices, 49
Voice Handicap Index-10 (VHI-10), 14, 24, 57, 65, 77
Voice therapy, 57
Voice turbulence index (VTI), 23, 32

Y
Yellowish discoloration, 54

GPSR Compliance

The European Union's (EU) General Product Safety Regulation (GPSR) is a set of rules that requires consumer products to be safe and our obligations to ensure this.

If you have any concerns about our products, you can contact us on ProductSafety@springernature.com

In case Publisher is established outside the EU, the EU authorized representative is:

Springer Nature Customer Service Center GmbH
Europaplatz 3
69115 Heidelberg, Germany

Batch number: 10731397

Printed by Printforce, the Netherlands